The Inside Out Diet

4 Weeks to Natural Weight Loss, Total Body Health, and Radiance

Cathy Wong, N.D. C.N.S.

with Recipes by Sabra Ricci

BICENTENNIAL
1807
WILEY
2007
BICENTENNIAL

John Wiley & Sons, Inc.

Published by John Wiley & Sons, Inc., Hoboken, New Jersey
Published simultaneously in Canada

All art by Tim Fedak; art copyright © 2007 Cathy Wong, N.D.

Wiley Bicentennial Logo: Richard J. Pacifico

Design and composition by Navta Associates, Inc.

The information contained in this book is not intended to serve as a replacement for professional medical advice. Any use of the information in this book is at the reader's discretion. The author and the publisher specifically disclaim any and all liability arising directly or indirectly from the use or application of any information contained in this book. A health care professional should be consulted regarding your specific situation.

For general information about our other products and services, please contact our Customer Care Department within the United States at (800) 762-2974, outside the United States at (317) 572-3993 or fax (317) 572-4002.

Wiley also publishes its books in a variety of electronic formats. Some content that appears in print may not be available in electronic books. For more information about Wiley products, visit our web site at www.wiley.com.

Library of Congress Cataloging-in-Publication Data:

Wong, Catherine.
   The inside out diet : 4 weeks to natural weight loss, total body health, and radiance / Catherine Wong ; with recipes by Sabra Ricci.
      p. cm.
   Includes bibliographical references and index.
   ISBN 978-0-471-79211-6 (cloth)
1. Weight loss. 2. Nutrition. 3. Naturopathy. I. Ricci, Sabra. II. Title.
   RM222.2W585 2007
   613.2'5—dc22

                                                                  2006036215

Printed in the United States of America

10   9   8   7   6   5   4   3   2   1

For Thomas

Contents

Acknowledgments

I would like to thank my husband, Thomas—you have been so support-ive, helpful, and patient during the long hours I spent working on this book. Thanks to my parents, Peter and Jacqueline Wong, for their unwa-vering support, ideas, and encouragement throughout the years, and Harold and Erna Redekopp, for their love and interest in my work.

I'm also thankful for the love and support of the rest of my family—my brother, Richard Wong, my sister Christine Wong, my sister-in-law Tannis Redekopp and her family, and all of my uncles, aunts, and cousins.

Megathanks to my literary agent, Susan Crawford, who has been a great source of guidance throughout the writing and production of this book.

My deepest thanks and appreciation to Christel Winkler, my editor at John Wiley & Sons, and to Tom Miller, Juliet Grames, Kimberly Monroe-Hill, Catherine Revland, and the rest of the talented team at Wiley.

Very special thanks to Sabra Ricci, for your commitment to excellence and dedication to your work and to this book. You took my nutritional the-ories and guidelines and translated them into the most delicious, satisfy-ing, and practical recipes.

Terri Trespicio, I can't thank you enough for enthusiastically, tirelessly, and quickly reading the final manuscript and helping to shape this infor-mation to make it more practical and readable. Leah Feldon, my heartfelt thanks for reading and commenting on an early draft, and for your advice and kindness during the more challenging moments. Sam Horn, you were instrumental in transforming an idea into a solid book proposal during the Maui Writers Retreat and for helping me connect with Susan.

I am indebted to the many colleagues from whom I have learned so much throughout my career: Jeffrey Bland, Ph.D., Peter Bennett, N.D., Burton Goldberg, Tim Tanaka, Ph.D., Barry Sears, Ph.D., Joseph Mercola, D.O., Ann Louise Gittleman, C.N.S., Ph.D., and Mitch Gaynor, M.D.

I would also like to thank Tim Fedak for the clear and simple illustrations in the book. Elliott and Esamor Krash and Sabra Ricci and Ally Pennebaker, for generously opening their homes to me during my stay in Maui, the Maui Writers Group for sharing their suggestions, Annie Nisula at Stanton Crenshaw Communications, Pearl Small at the Certification Board for Nutritional Specialists, and Gary MacDonald, for your help on the Amherst Island homefront.

To the whole crew at About.com—my editors Marc Lallanilla and Joy Victory, Marjorie Martin, Kate Grossman, M.D., Scott Meyer, Avram Piltch, Michael Daecher, Matt Law, Jessica Luterman, Lydia West, Lisa Langsdorf, Gina Carey, Eric Hanson, Crystal Marcus-Kanesaka, and the rest of the team—I appreciate your support throughout the years. Special thanks to Mary Shomon of Thyroid.about.com—you are an inspiration and have been so generous with your help. Thanks also to Shereen Jegvtig, D.C., C.N.S., of Nutrition.about.com, Paige Waehner of Exercise.about.com, Robin Elise Weiss of Pregnancy.about.com, Phylameana lila Desy of Healing.about.com, and the rest of my fellow guides, who are smart, talented, and committed writers and advocates.

Special kudos to Jon Evans, for his advice and perspective and for good-naturedly participating in impromptu taste testings, and to Holly Harben, for always being a ready source of great ideas. Thanks to Erik Rosen and Michelle Cooper, for giving feedback on the manuscript, and to Sara Collings, Du La, N.D., Jonah Lusis, N.D., Lisa Liberatore, Vic Sehgal, Rishma Walji Ajmera, N.D., Ann Nakajima, N.D., Davina and Matt Small, Erica and Ted Howell, Vivian Leung and Michael Innis, Eric Swan, John Thacker, Mark Gillingham, Irene and James Paxton, Julie Hogan and Briscoe Rodgers, and the many other friends who listened, brainstormed, helped, or just cheered me on during the writing of this book.

And finally, thanks to my clients, whom I have had the honor of working with, and my readers, whose e-mails, insights, and enthusiasm are a continuous source of inspiration.

May you all live well!

Introduction

When I was in college at the University of Toronto and struggling with my own weight (I gained twenty pounds over four years) and constantly in a rush and under deadline, I took shortcuts to get through the day. I'd skip breakfast, suck down coffee after coffee, skip lunch, and then, by day's end, despite my best efforts to resist, I'd surrender to the siren call of the fast-food restaurant on my way home and hungrily devour a burger and fries, scolding myself the whole time. *I blew it again*, I'd say. This would be followed by a vow to go for a run as soon as I got home—a plan that was soon forgotten once I sat down to read the paper and found myself fast asleep by ten o'clock, only to wake up the next day and do it all over again.

My rationale was simple: sure, I knew that my eating habits weren't great, but, I argued, I loved food too much! Health food was too bland for me. And besides, I worked hard all day and deserved to treat myself. After college, when I started training to become a nutritionist and a naturopathic doctor, I found myself surrounded by people who were well hydrated, avoided coffee, and ate veggies and drank green drinks. It was a shock. I remember thinking, *I could never do that*. It didn't seem appetizing.

I continued with my old ways, skipping meals, not eating enough vegetables, grabbing muffins, pizza, and bagels on the go, but gradually felt worse and worse. Then one day, I went in for my annual physical and was told that my cholesterol was borderline high—and I was only twenty-four! This really hit home since my grandparents had died from heart disease and diabetes. That night, I lay in bed thinking that no matter how hard it would be, I had to try to break this cycle.

The next day, I began a liver-cleansing diet. At first, I must admit, I was a bit skeptical about what it could do for me. I rarely drank alcohol, didn't do drugs, and didn't smoke—how much cleansing would my liver need? But I went ahead anyway. Almost immediately, I started to feel better. My digestion improved. My energy came back. My cholesterol and weight came down. I hadn't felt like this in years. I felt like I was waking up again.

Now, of course it does take some work and dedication to break old habits and fit new things into your lifestyle, and sometimes I lapsed back into my old ways because eating healthy day in and day out seemed impossible—especially when I was eating foods I was unaccustomed to. But as my tastes evolved, I began to really appreciate these foods because I felt really good when I ate them. My energy soared. I felt positive and vibrant, and people commented, for the first time, about the healthy glow I had. And the best part about it? I realized that as long as I maintained healthy habits and included the right foods, I could still enjoy any foods I loved, as long as I did it in moderation. It took a real commitment to myself and my health, but as I quickly discovered, it was worth it.

Many of you already know me as the guide to alternative medicine at About.com, one of the most popular and trusted Web sites for practical information. According to the World Health Organization, 158 million of the adult population use alternative medicine in the United States. For the last seven years, I've reviewed the latest in diet and health research, and written hundreds of articles for readers around the world who count on me for my scientific evidence, real-life experience, and a down-to-earth approach.

When I posted basic information about this type of diet on the site, overnight it became one of the most popular pages. People couldn't get enough of it, and I received thousands of e-mails from readers everywhere, asking me when I was going to write a book and give them the full plan. This is it!

Today, as a nutritionist and a naturopathic doctor who uses herbal medicine, acupuncture, lifestyle counseling, relaxation therapies, and other natural therapies to create individualized treatment plans, I see clients who have tried everything to lose weight. And I mean everything. South Beach. Atkins. The Grapefruit Diet. The Mediterranean Diet. The Zone. Weight Watchers. The Three-Hour Diet. Calorie counting. Even prescription drugs. Do these things help them lose weight? Sometimes, but it often doesn't last. And soon they're back at square one, having lost little more than their resolve. In fact, some of my clients suffer such dramatic fluctuations in weight that they simply keep different sets of clothing to suit their shifting sizes.

All these trial-and-error techniques have taught them some valuable lessons. They've learned that simply cutting calories won't work; they end up hungry, tired, and worse—obsessed with the food they can't have. They've learned that quantifying your food by measuring every unit is painstaking, joyless, and not viable as a long-term solution. The prescription drugs have uncomfortable, sometimes horrible side effects. And maintaining a multisize wardrobe can be expensive.

Clients come to me frustrated, upset, beaten down, apologetic. Some look resigned, others embarrassed. Some fight back tears. And they've come to me with the very last shred of hope they can muster. Unfortunately, difficulty with weight loss is rarely their only problem. The struggle with weight often comes coupled with other health problems, too: high blood pressure, hot flashes, fatigue, arthritis, chronic stress, indigestion, high cholesterol, sports injuries, skin problems, insomnia, and depression, to name a few. Many of these conditions, including weight, I've found, can be helped by addressing certain underlying problems like hormonal imbalance, essential fatty acid deficiency, chronic inflammation, inadequate diet, chemical exposure, stress, and food intolerances, which all involve the liver.

I take a holistic approach to health in my practice, paying special attention to the role nutrition plays in our health. Many of the people I see have been told by doctors that there is nothing wrong with them, even though they know in their gut there is. The truth is, 65 percent of adults in the United States are overweight or obese, and most North Americans regularly lose and regain weight. According to a report by the Institute of Medicine, over two-thirds of the weight a person loses will be regained within a year and almost all within five years. Whether you are trying to lose that last fifteen pounds or drop the fifty you gained back, the fact remains that gaining and losing and then gaining weight again can take a serious toll on your health.

The big selling point for most fad diets is how rapidly weight loss occurs. In this book, you'll learn what my clients already know and have experienced firsthand—that a healthy liver, while often overlooked and certainly underappreciated, is critical to maintaining a healthy weight. And when its health is compromised, our most important metabolic functions, involving our thyroid, insulin, and other hormones, grind to a halt—as does our ability to lose weight. Fad diets that encourage rapid weight loss cause a rapid influx of fats and toxins to your poor liver, over-taxing it and thus rendering it less capable of doing its job.

Unlike most diet books that take aim at food as the enemy, this plan helps you see food differently—as a wonderful and natural tool for heal-ing and weight loss. My clients, who have successfully lost and kept off their weight, know that the only effective weight loss happens when they shift their focus from eating for loss (what not to eat) to eating to gain—health, energy, and a sense of well-being, that is. You might be thinking that this doesn't sound like dieting, because it's not. And that's why it works.

Once my clients started eating foods that would improve the health of their liver, the weight began to come off, and continued to, without hit-ting that plateau. Not only that, but they began to feel energized and pas-sionate about living again! For many of them it was the first time they were eating to have more energy and vitality, to control their stress, and to reduce pain—rather than eating (or not eating) to fit into smaller-size pants. Although I don't believe in a magic bullet, I quickly realized that this diet was as close to one as you could find.

What to Expect

When my clients first start this plan, most begin to feel better after only a few days. By the end of the first week, they feel lighter, cleaner, and more energized. And while you may experience the effects of the plan rather quickly, it's not a quick-fix diet. The real benefits come in the longer term with sustained weight loss and a vast improvement in your health and well-being.

The first week is the most restrictive part of the plan, aimed at elimi-nating unhealthy cravings, improving insulin and leptin sensitivity, restor-ing hormonal balance, correcting your metabolism, and cleansing the colon and liver to open the pathways for sustained fat loss. Think of it as spring cleaning for the body—at any time of the year.

After this week is over, you'll bring back certain foods into your diet in the first week of step 2, but not haphazardly. Many diets unnecessarily restrict foods. With this diet, you'll find out which foods are particularly problematic for you and only limit those. You'll continue with step 2 for another two weeks (although many people choose to stay in step 2 until they've reached their goal weight), enjoying a wide variety of delicious and satisfying dishes, such as Rosemary Grilled Lamb with Goat Cheese, Roasted Beets, Red Onion, and Warm Watercress; Beef Tenderloin Scalloppini; and Mixed Baby Greens with Blood Oranges, Almonds, and Pomegranates.

Then in step 3, you'll do what I do and what my clients do to stay healthy and maintain your success: follow your plan five days a week and then indulge in some of the other foods you like (in moderation, of course) on the other two days. This solves the problem of boredom. It also keeps your metabolism revved so you don't regain any of the weight. This is your plan for life. And because you're not permanently restricting yourself from any foods, you'll never "mess up."

How much weight will you lose? Remember, faster isn't better, as rapid weight loss can take a serious toll on your health (despite the praise actresses get for losing weight the fastest). Losing weight fast throws a wrench into your weight loss by causing metabolic slowdown and releasing chemicals that scream "Stop!" to your body. This in turn can promote the formation of gallstones and liver disease. In an age of extreme makeovers and instant fixes, it's hard to accept that changing your lifestyle and making long-term adjustments can take some time. But trust me, it pays off. Big time. My clients lose one to two pounds a week, and these are pounds that they keep off.

How This Diet Will Help You

People on this diet have experienced life-changing results, from those who feel like they've lost ten years off their life rather than just ten pounds, to those like my client Tony, whose long-standing sports injury resolved after several weeks on this diet. Specifically, it has been developed to achieve the following:

- Help you lose weight safely, continuously, and permanently
- Improve liver function and decrease fatty liver

- Restore insulin and leptin sensitivity
- Improve cholesterol and triglyceride levels
- Eliminate unhealthy cravings
- Decrease risk factors for heart disease
- Re-establish hormonal balance
- Improve overall health

Although my priority is your inner health, people who try this diet also notice an improvement in their appearance. In contrast, when people try fad diets, they often say they think they look older, which is due to inflammation and toxin release that damages collagen, blood vessels, and other body tissues. The difference between the wrong diet and the right one is noticeable and makes itself evident in every aspect of their health.

A Lovable and Livable Diet

There are many reasons why this is a plan you will find irresistible, even in the long term.

- This diet is not just about eating less, it's about eating the right foods for your liver. As you're about to learn, the liver is involved in weight loss, and maximizing and supporting liver function with the right foods will allow you to lose weight safely and permanently.
- It is based on whole foods. The average American diet is filled with high-calorie foods made with bad fats, sugar, and salt, all manufactured to make us crave and overeat them. "Diet" foods often aren't much better. Many are filled with chemicals and aren't as nutrient-rich as we think they are. The Inside Out Diet emphasizes the goodness of nature. It will reacquaint your taste buds with delightful, satisfying natural flavors, and pretty soon you will notice a remarkable change—you will no longer crave addictive foods that aren't good for you and will intuitively reach for healthy foods.
- It's a realistic long-term plan. I won't give you a diet that lasts several weeks or months and then say "see ya!" I won't leave you with a diet that keeps you on a strict leash 24/7—or else—for the rest of your life. Life isn't about boot camp. This diet is a way of life, allowing you to eventually eat what you like, in moderation.
- It will work for your busy life. I made sure this was doable and would

fit in with hectic schedules. Although it initially requires you to make changes, once you get into the flow, it's quite simple.

- You won't need to take ten billion diet pills a day. I *will* suggest certain supplements, such as essential fatty acids, but they will be part of a minimal core plan. Instead of relying on supplements, we will take advantage of the healing properties of food. People with certain health conditions, however, may require further support.

- The recipes are delicious and satisfying. The recipes in this book were created by chef Sabra Ricci, a chef to the stars and a caterer on the island of Maui. A graduate of the California Culinary Academy in San Francisco, Sabra is renowned for her healthy, delectable menus. She created these recipes to fit the guidelines of this diet, and I have no doubt you'll enjoy them.

Who Shouldn't Try This Diet

Nothing is right for everyone. Although this diet is safe for most men and women, reactions can vary. It's always a good idea to consult your doctor before trying anything new, especially if you take medication or have a health condition. In particular, people with kidney disease, severe liver disease, hyperthyroidism, autoimmune disease, eating disorders, cancer, terminal illness, certain genetic diseases, and other chronic conditions should not try this diet, or should do so only under the supervision of their primary care provider. Pregnant or nursing women or children should not try this diet.

Getting Started

Because the focus of this approach to eating and weight loss is internally, rather than externally, focused, it's important to learn a little about how your body works (in particular your liver) so that you can work with it to lose weight, instead of against it. I recommend reading the following chapters to give you an overview before you begin to put it into action. If you are eager to get started, however, you can flip to the appropriate pages to find the food lists, guidelines, menu plans, and recipes right now.

Part I

The Key to Natural Weight Loss

1

The Liver Link

Is life worth living? It all depends on the liver.
—PHILOSOPHER WILLIAM JAMES

My client Barb, a nurse for twenty years, had been struggling with her weight for as long as she could remember. A chronic yo-yo dieter, she tried diet after diet with little success. Long hours, hospital cafeteria food, and a smoking habit didn't help, but the fact remained that while she could lose weight in the short term, the pounds would creep back. To say she was skeptical of any new diet was putting it mildly.

Barb came to me because she was experiencing low energy, joint pain, and indigestion. When her doctor couldn't find a cause, he sent her home with painkillers. But that didn't sit well with Barb; she knew there had to be a better way. During our hourlong visit, I explained to Barb that certain foods were contributing to her problem. I pointed out that the types of meat and fish, cheese, and diet snacks she ate, and the bagels and breakfast cereals she had for breakfast, were contributing to her symptoms. And while I was not recommending that Barb switch to a vegetarian diet (nor do I think this is the answer for everyone), I did recommend foods that would address the underlying cause—an overtaxed liver.

Four weeks after starting this diet, she returned to my office. She reported that she began to feel better almost overnight. Her skin looked better, and she felt calmer, more rested, and energized. But what surprised her most was how she had lost weight—without even feeling hungry. "Everyone at work wants to try it," she said, "but when they asked me why it would help with weight loss, I didn't know quite how to explain it. What does my liver have to do with my weight?"

"Everything," I said. The liver is the secret to weight loss and health, and one of the most important missing pieces of the weight-loss puzzle. If you aren't eating foods that support liver function, you could be placing further burden on it and keeping yourself from losing weight.

Your Liver and Its Connection to Your Overall Health

Have you ever felt overworked, overburdened, and underappreciated? If your liver could talk, that's what it would say. The word "liver" is derived from the Old English word meaning "for life"—a name it surely deserves. As your body's main processing plant and an incredible multitasker, involved in over five hundred vital functions, your liver has more to do with well-being than you might think. This wedge-shaped organ, located under your ribs on your right side above the stomach, is your largest internal organ, weighing about 3 percent of your body's total weight. Almost all metabolic activities and body functions are dependent on the liver in some way, and that's why it's centrally located in our bodies, allowing it to easily communicate with our other body parts. It's also the only organ that can regenerate itself if damaged.

The liver's many functions include:

- Helping us metabolize the fats, protein, and carbohydrates we eat
- Creating proteins needed for healthy blood cells and the immune system
- Making cell membranes
- Producing hormones
- Facilitating the absorption of essential vitamins
- Filtering and breaking down all unwanted compounds produced during metabolism
- Removing chemicals and bacteria from blood

Although the liver is quite capable of doing its job, the diets we eat—not to mention the ever-increasing levels of chemicals in our environment—can push it to capacity. When this happens, the liver has to work overtime to detoxify the body, leaving it less able to carry out its many other roles—resulting in what is called an overburdened liver.

And because it is involved in the formation and breakdown of mood-affecting hormones and neurotransmitters (chemicals that help transmit messages between nerve cells), the liver also influences your emotions. If the liver isn't functioning well, these chemicals can be thrown out of balance, causing changes in our mood.

This connection between the liver and mood is well known and respected in many ancient medical traditions. In traditional Chinese medicine (TCM), it is believed that anger stems from stagnant liver energy, which can also cause conditions such as premenstrual syndrome, diabetes, headaches, muscle and joint pain, digestive problems, and vision disorders. In ayurveda, the traditional medicine of India, anger and aggression are also associated with the fire element and the liver. In France today, when someone is not feeling well, it's called *mal au foie*, or "sick in the liver."

Ancient cultures have also known for centuries that food affects liver health, which is why the prescribed treatment for the liver in TCM and ayurveda often centers around diet. Even in Germany today, it's not uncommon for physicians to recommend herbal liver remedies such as artichoke for people with high cholesterol and chronic ailments. In fact, artichoke is one of the top-selling herbs in Germany.

Wait a minute, you may be asking yourself. If the liver is so darned important, why do we hear so little about it? It's true that the liver's central role in health and weight loss has only recently been recognized and appreciated. Hepatology, the branch of medicine concerned with the functions and disorders of the liver, has only existed as a medical specialty for the last fifty years. And, as recently as twenty years ago, there were still relatively few treatments for liver disorders. One reason is that conventional lab tests often miss an overburdened liver in its early stages. Another is that symptoms tend to be nonspecific, such as fatigue—or they turn up in parts of the body you might not expect, such as the skin.

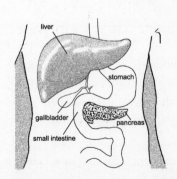

The liver and other internal organs.

One of the clear signs that the liver is overloaded is that it can't process fat properly but instead stores it. This condition, called fatty liver, is related to obesity and diabetes and can even lead to serious liver disease. Although liver diseases were once believed to affect only a very small number of people, in the past decade, studies have shown that one in four people have fatty liver. It's shocking, I know, but most liver problems are attributable to years of eating the wrong foods and our modern lifestyle, which leaves our poor livers struggling to keep up.

Certain risk factors can increase the likelihood of having a tired and toxic liver. The more factors you have, the greater your risk. Any of the following can complicate the problem.

- High fat or sugar intake
- Overly cutting back on carbohydrates
- Not getting enough protein
- Diets high in refined carbohydrates
- Consuming too few calories
- Not getting enough fiber
- Eating certain fish or seafood regularly
- Diets lacking in certain nutrients
- Eating too much bad fat and not enough good fat
- Not eating enough vegetables
- Drinking alcohol regularly
- Smoking cigarettes
- Relying on processed diet foods or fast food
- Certain prescription and nonprescription drugs
- Insulin resistance

Liver Self-Test: Is an Overworked Liver Sabotaging Your Weight?

While there is no single lab or diagnostic test to clearly and definitively diagnose an overburdened liver, there are some telltale signs that may indicate your liver has more than it can handle. Keep in mind that any of these symptoms on their own do not mean you have a serious liver problem. In fact, some of them may be signs of another issue altogether. If you experience persistent symptoms, however, or several of them in combination, I recommend bringing them to your doctor's attention.

The following are signs that indicate you may need to resuscitate your liver. Check the ones that apply to you.

Weight

- ☐ Excessive weight gain, especially around the abdomen
- ☐ Cravings for sweet, starchy, or fatty foods
- ☐ Constant hunger
- ☐ Difficulty losing weight

Energy

- ☐ Fatigue
- ☐ Feeling groggy in the morning
- ☐ Feeling the urge to lie down frequently

Digestion

- ☐ Constipation
- ☐ Heartburn
- ☐ Bad breath
- ☐ Abdominal bloating or gas
- ☐ Bitter taste in the mouth

Mental/Emotional

- ☐ Irritability or anger, tendency to fly off the handle
- ☐ Depression
- ☐ Negative thoughts
- ☐ Mood swings
- ☐ Poor concentration or brain "fog"
- ☐ Always feeling stressed

Pain

- ☐ Ache in the upper right abdomen
- ☐ Headaches related to tension or stress
- ☐ Joint pain

Hormonal

- ☐ Benign breast cysts
- ☐ Premenstrual syndrome with irritability
- ☐ Infertility

Skin

- ☐ Dark undereye circles
- ☐ Acne

☐ Skin rash
☐ Poor skin tone
☐ Spider veins
☐ Dark patches of skin pigmentation
☐ Itching
☐ Psoriasis
☐ Frequent bruising
☐ Hemorrhoids
☐ Premature aging

General
☐ Body odor
☐ Excess body heat or hot flushes
☐ Water retention
☐ Dry eyes
☐ Itchy, red eyes
☐ Weak tendons, ligaments, muscles
☐ Stools that float
☐ Light-colored stools

It's quite a list. But again, keep in mind that these are generalized symptoms and that you need not suffer all of them in order to experience real benefits from a liver-cleansing diet plan. And for most people, an overburdened liver can be healed and improved with the proper diet and care. You can take simple steps to restore your liver to a vital, optimally functioning dynamo—as early as today! Once you do, you'll not only begin to drop pounds and reverse the above symptoms but also will start to feel better overall.

But first things first. You're probably curious about how your liver can help you lose weight. Let's take a look at how your liver is connected to weight loss.

The Liver's Role in Weight Loss

Your Liver Regulates Blood Sugar

When we talk about insulin resistance, we tend to focus on the pancreas, and rightly so, since the pancreas produces insulin; the liver, however, plays a major and often overlooked role in carbohydrate metabolism. The liver stores and releases glucose in order to control our blood sugar at all times; it also produces glucose from other nutrients. When we have more glucose than we need, the hormone insulin is released, which tells the liver to convert the excess glucose to glycogen, a form in which glucose can be stored. If you then skip lunch and your blood sugar dwindles, it's the liver's job to break down glycogen and convert it back to glucose for fuel.

When the liver gets overloaded—as is the case for many of us—your ability to properly control your blood sugar can become impaired. And if the liver isn't properly doing its job as a blood sugar regulator, it can lead to weight gain, cravings for sweets and starchy foods, fatigue, constant hunger, diabetes, inflammation, and premature aging.

Your Liver Makes and Burns Fat

The liver is the main site where the excess carbohydrates we eat are converted into fatty acids and ultimately, triglycerides, which are stored in fat cells. It is also the place where triglyceride fat, along with protein, can be broken down to provide an alternative source of energy when glucose is unavailable.

Your Liver Helps You Absorb Omega Fatty Acids

Your liver produces about a quart of bile each day from bile acids, cholesterol, bilirubin, electrolytes, and lecithin. Once released by the liver, most of this soupy, greenish-brown fluid travels through special ducts to the gallbladder, where it's stored and concentrated for when your body needs it to digest fats.

The role of bile in the body is to absorb dietary fat. Whenever we eat anything containing fat, such as nuts, meat, fish, or cookies, the presence of fat in the intestines triggers the release of bile from the gallbladder into the small intestine to help digest the fat. Bile acts like a detergent, breaking apart the large droplets of fat to smaller droplets so they can be absorbed. Bile also helps absorb vitamins A, D, E, and K, known as the fat-soluble vitamins, and helps with iron and vitamin B12 absorption and the conversion of beta-carotene to vitamin A.

Two types of fat, known collectively as the essential fatty acids (omega-3 and omega-6) because the body cannot produce them on its own and needs to obtain them from food, have a critical role in weight loss. Omega-3 fats appear to help us:

- Raise our metabolic rate and burn fat. Omega-3 fats have also been found to reduce the size and number of fat cells, especially in the abdomen.
- Make cell membranes permeable and fluid so cells can properly communicate with one another
- Improve the sensitivity of hormones insulin and leptin
- Prevent gallstone formation during weight loss
- Reduce excess fat in the liver

Research shows that a certain kind of omega-6, called gamma linolenic acid, or GLA, also helps us shed pounds, by decreasing body fat, helping the body burn calories, and reducing the amount of calories consumed.

Most of us don't get enough omegas in our diets. To compound the problem, when we carry extra weight or go on a diet without simultaneously detoxing the liver, the all-important flow of bile slows down. Without enough bile flowing into the intestines, we are unable to absorb the essential fatty acids critical for weight loss and health. The result is weight gain, dry, scaly skin, brittle nails and hair, poor concentration and memory, and may eventually lead to insomnia, depression, heart disease, inflammation, and insulin resistance.

Your Liver Regulates Cholesterol

The liver controls how much cholesterol we have. Although many people think of cholesterol as something we get through our diet, in fact, our liver manufactures most of our cholesterol. It also makes the lipoproteins, including high-density lipoprotein (HDL), low-density lipoprotein (LDL), and very-low-density lipoprotein (VLDL), that transport cholesterol around the body.

Most people think of cholesterol as something they don't want too much of. While high cholesterol is a risk factor for heart disease, cholesterol is not all bad. It's an important and necessary component of all our cells. It's also the raw material used to make bile acids and steroid hormones, such as estrogen, progesterone, testosterone, dehydroepiandrosterone (DHEA), and cortisol, which help us maintain hormonal balance.

If there is an excess of cholesterol, it gets absorbed by bile, then excreted in the stools. But if there is too much cholesterol and not enough bile acids and lecithin to keep bile fluid, bile can become too thick and form gallstones. In fact, gallstones are fairly common and often go undiagnosed in people who are overweight as well as in those trying to lose weight.

Your Liver Balances Key Weight-Loss Hormones

Another key function of the liver is to regulate the production and inactivation of many of the body's hormones, including estrogen and cortisol and the neurotransmitters serotonin and dopamine. If the liver isn't functioning at full tilt, there may be signs of hormonal imbalance.

Cortisol

One of the most important hormones involved in the stress response is the hormone cortisol. It is produced by the adrenal glands, two nut-size glands that sit on top of the kidneys. Elevated cortisol levels disrupt our body's balanced state, resulting in weight gain in the abdomen, constant hunger pangs and cravings, elevated blood sugar, widespread inflammation, fluid retention, muscle weakness, insulin resistance, and high blood pressure.

Case in point: my client Carol, a sales consultant, walked into my office one day and collapsed into a chair. "I hate my job," she said. "I sit in my office at the computer and on the phone all day working like crazy to make these sales, under constant pressure from my manager. Sometimes it almost feels like I'm going to have a heart attack. Plus, my neck and shoulders are so tense, they're killing me. I've gotten into a habit of keeping candy bars and crackers in my desk to snack on when I don't have time to get out for lunch. I know they're not good for me, but sometimes, in a day when everything seems to be going wrong, they're the only thing that's right. I know I should be more disciplined, but I don't have the mental energy to be vigilant. My willpower's shot."

Like Carol, many of us live with unremitting pressure. What's becoming increasingly apparent is that although our bodies can deal with short-lived stresses, many of us live with continual stress, and the sustained elevations in cortisol take a huge toll on our weight and our health. There are three ways chronic stress can affect your weight.

1. *Stubborn belly fat.* George Chrousos, M.D., at the National Institutes of Health, and Pamela Peeke, M.D., were among the first to research

the relationship between stress and abdominal fat. It turns out that stress causes a cascade of responses that encourages the body to store fat deep in the belly around the vital organs. Abdominal fat is very sensitive to cortisol and has a higher density of cortisol receptors. When they get turned on by stress, the belly becomes a virtual fat factory.

Why the abdomen? Fat here can be quickly converted to energy. Because the brain thinks that it and the body are under continual siege when stressed, abdominal fat stores can provide a quick source of energy during the long spell of stress. This hardwired response enabled our hunter-gatherer ancestors to survive when food was scarce by giving their bodies immediate access to this excess energy store. The problem is that nowadays it's primarily psychological stress that threatens us. When you are faced with looming deadlines, a domineering boss, money issues, marital problems, or emotional issues in the past or present, you don't need the extra abdominal fat.

A fascinating Yale study demonstrated that people who tend to get more stressed and release more cortisol also have more belly fat. Researchers looked at forty-one women who were overweight, half with abdominal fat and the other half with fat centered around their thighs. They gave the women six stressful tasks to do, including solving math problems under a time limit, making speeches, and solving puzzles. Their cortisol levels were then measured. The researchers found that the women with abdominal fat released more cortisol than the women who stored fat in their hips.

2. *Constant hunger.* Although temporary stress can sometimes take away our appetite, when we are chronically stressed, we become hungry. Again, it's a programmed physiological response that enabled the early humans to survive. Cortisol ensures that we have fuel in a form that can be quickly converted into blood sugar to give us energy and replenish the sugar we might burn. The preferred fuel? Carbohydrates. That's why when we are under stress, we crave junk food like sugar, muffins, cookies, cake, chocolate, and other sweets we know aren't good for us. And exactly how does cortisol turn on cravings? Neurobiologist Sara Leibowitz from Rockefeller University has found that cortisol turns on a hunger-promoting brain chemical called neuropeptide Y, which is produced in the hypothalamus, making us crave sweets and other carbohydrate-rich foods. Cortisol also appears to reduce levels of adiponectin, an appetite-suppressing hormone.

If the stress is chronic and involves nothing more than sitting at your desk, you don't need all this fuel. But cortisol still sends out its message, resulting in constant hunger pangs. The result: we eat more than we need and gain weight.

Elissa Epel, Ph.D., and colleagues at the University of California at San Francisco, demonstrated this connection between high cortisol and hunger and snacking when they found that women with high cortisol levels eat more food, particularly sweets. They gave fifty-nine women, with an average age of thirty-six, a challenging task to do but not enough time to complete it. Each woman's stress level was assessed by taking cortisol readings and asking her to rate her mood. Afterward, the women went to a quiet room and were allowed to read or listen to music. Snacks were placed in front of them, although they weren't pressured to eat. Women who were the most stressed and had the highest cortisol level snacked more, particularly on sweets. What does this mean for you? On the days you feel pressured and pressed for time, you'll most likely find yourself reaching for food. Until you address the stress, each day will be a battle to fight these temptations.

3. *Blood sugar rush.* When we are under chronic stress, the metabolic derangement that ensues inhibits the normal process of insulin release and sugar uptake, keeping sugar in the bloodstream longer than normal. Blood sugar levels remain elevated, which damages tissue and can lead to premature aging. To make matters worse, insulin further increases as it desperately tries to rein in blood sugar.

Peter Vitaliano, Ph.D., and colleagues at the University of Washington, demonstrated the link between stress and diabetes. They compared forty-seven people who were caregivers for their spouses with Alzheimer's disease to seventy-seven people who were noncaregivers. As we'd expect, the researchers found that the caregivers felt more stress, depression, fear, and lack of control. But they also discovered that cortisol, glucose, and insulin levels were higher in the caregivers compared to the noncaregivers, putting them at a higher risk for developing diabetes.

The role of chronic stress as a trigger may partially explain why diabetes rates are soaring in people at younger ages: the incidence of type 2 diabetes increased 33 percent between 1990 and 1998 in the United States, with a 76 percent jump in the incidence of diabetes in people in their thirties.

Serotonin

Involved in sleep, mood, and appetite, serotonin is our inner Zen master, keeping us calm and content. The liver and digestive tract are involved in making serotonin and breaking it down. If the liver is overloaded, it can't do this properly. Signs that serotonin is out of balance include the following.

- *Continuously eating or bingeing on sugar and other carbohydrates.* If you have low serotonin, you may unwittingly be reaching for carbohydrates as your body's way of trying to restore serotonin levels. In the early 1970s, in an MIT lab, neuroscientist Richard Wurtman and psychologist John Fernstrom were the first to discover that carbohydrate consumption triggered a biochemical chain of reactions resulting in higher serotonin levels. The foods we tend to reach for—cookies, muffins, chocolate, doughnuts, and other sweets—temporarily raise serotonin. We feel better, but it's short-lived. Eventually the effect wears off, serotonin levels fall, and the hunger returns. The result is weight gain.

  Study after study has linked low serotonin with increased appetite, overeating, and obesity in both animals and humans. Animals with low serotonin will continue to binge on food, even if they're given a warning cue to shock them or if they're actually given a shock. Nothing will stop an animal from bingeing if its brain senses that it's deprived of serotonin.

- *Poor body image.* Serotonin influences the way we perceive and think about ourselves. For instance, when serotonin levels start to fall, we may become unhappy with the way we look, no matter what size we are. We may look in the mirror and only see flaws. We might even start obsessing about food and everything we eat. Our mood may rapidly deteriorate. Self-esteem may also wane.

- *Obsessing about food.* When serotonin levels fall, a vicious cycle can be set in motion because the more we diet, the lower our serotonin levels drop, and the harder we try to diet. We become overly critical of ourselves, obsessed with thoughts or behaviors we can't seem to shut off. We scrutinize our eating habits and become

Telltale Signs of Low Serotonin Levels

If you feel yourself starting to get fixated on counting calories, carbohydrates, or eating in general while dieting, your serotonin levels may be dropping too low.

hypervigilant about our food intake, obsessed with calories, and unhealthily focused on attaining the perfect body. Our thoughts can also become rigid and inflexible. One common complaint I hear from clients is that they get so caught up in the "rights" and "wrongs" of the diet that when they break these self-imposed "rules," they feel that they've failed and decide to give up altogether. So if you've ever felt those diets you tried were literally messing with your head, you were right. It could have affected your serotonin levels.

- *Eating at night.* Depleted serotonin activates the urge to eat continuously in the evening. Someone with this pattern, called night-eating syndrome, might say, "I can't make it past seven p.m. I just start eating and can't stop." Or, "Every night I tell myself I'm not going to do it and the next thing you know I'm in the kitchen eating anything."

Over one quarter of people who are overweight experience this pattern, which also includes not being hungry in the morning, worsening mood and depression as the evening progresses, and an inability to get a good night's sleep.

Signs of Balanced Serotonin Levels	Signs of Serotonin Imbalance
Minimal reliance on sweets	Sugar and carbohydrate cravings
Positive outlook	Depression
Pleasant, easygoing disposition	Irritable, argumentative, hostile disposition
Self-confidence	Low self-esteem
Falling asleep easily, waking up refreshed	Insomnia, difficulty falling asleep or staying asleep
Feeling content and optimistic	Excessive worrying, moodiness
Cooperative nature	Insistence on having things your way
Normal experience of pain	Heightened pain sensitivity

These factors may cause your serotonin levels to drop:

- Chronic stress
- An imbalance of bacteria in the intestines
- Eating too few carbohydrates
- Artificial sweeteners
- Cigarette smoking
- Perimenopause and menopause

- Birth control pills
- Alcohol abuse

Dopamine

The neurotransmitter dopamine maintains a balance with serotonin to regulate appetite. A groundbreaking study led by Gene-Jack Wang, M.D., of the Department of Energy's Brookhaven lab, first demonstrated the link between dopamine and obesity. The researchers used brain imaging to show that the more a person weighed, the less dopamine there was in his or her brain. Like serotonin, it can get depleted with chronic stress. These are two of the ways dopamine affects weight.

1. *Causes overeating.* Dr. Wang's study was the first in a line of research suggesting that overeating is caused by the brain's desperate attempt to increase dopamine and get that satisfaction. We crave foods that are particularly good at increasing our endorphins—chemicals that make us feel good—such as ice cream, cheese, pudding, cheesecake, and other high-fat dairy, doughnuts, cakes, pastries, cookies, and chocolates.

2. *Decreases motivation and the ability to stick with a diet.* When we lose our enthusiasm for managing our food intake via dieting, we can become discouraged and even depressed. We feel like we've failed. In truth, low dopamine levels may be what's making you lose your drive and abandon your goals. Dopamine plays a critical role in our ability to plan, persevere, and stay focused. People with dopamine depletion are easily distracted when they see food and often find themselves constantly daydreaming about what they're going to eat next.

Dopamine also plays into our ability to compare the energy requirements of different actions. It is the reason why you may go with the easiest food option, even when it means breaking with your diet. So when the choice is, "Should I wash and cut up some veggie sticks or should I crack open one of those vanilla puddings I keep for the kids?" a dopamine-depleted person will find it particularly difficult to resist the pudding.

Your Liver Maintains Muscle Tone

The more lean muscle you have, the more fat and calories you burn, because muscle burns more calories than fat. Having more muscle also means that more glucose is taken up and burned rather than stored and turned into fat.

Muscle, just like skin, hair, teeth, and bones, is made up of protein, which in turn is composed of even smaller building blocks called amino acids. Our hormones, enzymes, and neurotransmitters are also made of protein. The liver has to assess what the body needs to make and then produce it. It breaks down old proteins and makes sure new ones are available.

Your Liver Gets Rid of Fattening Toxins

Your liver is truly the hardest-working kid on the block. In addition to all the functions I've described so far, almost everything that enters the body—everything we eat, breathe, or absorb through our skin—must be filtered and detoxified by the liver.

Put simply, the goal of liver detox is to convert toxins into a form that can easily be eliminated in stools or urine, preventing them from causing damage. Every minute, two quarts of unfiltered blood circulates to the liver via special blood vessels with small holes. These holes, called fenestrations, allow unwanted, potentially harmful substances to pass out of the bloodstream and into special liver cells that can dismantle these substances so they can be easily excreted from the body. Otherwise, they keep circulating and causing damage to our tissues and cells.

The process of detoxifying the liver is not unlike removing a stain from a shirt. The first step is to soak the shirt so that the stains will come out in the wash cycle. In step one of detox, unwanted substances are prepped so they can be excreted. A specialized enzyme system made up of fifty to one hundred enzymes, called cytochrome p450, alters the chemical structure to prepare these substances for elimination. Then comes the wash cycle, which lifts out the dirt and later drains it away during the spin cycle. Likewise, in step two of detox, liver cells attach a molecule to the unwanted substance that allows it to be flushed out of the body through urine (via the kidneys) or stools (via bile).

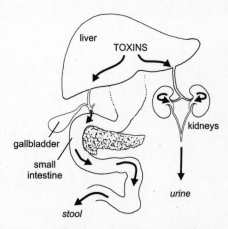

The liver's detoxification pathways.

I marvel at all the liver has to do. This role of the liver as detoxifier becomes critically important during weight loss. When we are exposed to toxins, such as mercury from fish or environmental pollutants, the body stores these toxins in fat cells. When those fat stores are broken down during weight loss—particularly rapid weight loss—the liver can be flooded with more toxins than it can handle, which in turn leaves it less able to maintain its other critical tasks. As you'll learn in the next chapter, this can interfere with our ability to lose weight. And because toxic overload affects every other system in the body as well, this can result in fatigue, allergies, inflammation, swollen glands, hormone imbalance, acne, headaches, an inability to digest and absorb foods, and other problems.

Now that you appreciate the liver's multitude of jobs, it's on to the next chapter, where we'll talk about the two concurrent blows to the liver that happen as a result of weight loss. In part III, you'll learn how to use the Inside Out Diet to prevent them and help you drop pounds, once and for all.

2

The Risks and Hazards of Dieting

I've been on a diet for two weeks, and all I've lost is two weeks.
—COMEDIAN TOTIE FIELDS

You may be familiar with this scenario: one morning you're watching your favorite talk show, flipping through a magazine, or browsing in a bookstore, and you find out about a new diet that's getting miraculous results. Look at those impressive before-and-after pictures! You begin the diet and are excited when you start dropping pounds. You tell a couple of friends and they try it, too, and also start to lose weight.

Then one morning it comes to a screeching halt. No matter what you do, the scale just won't budge, and you're wondering, "What am I doing wrong? If I could only discipline myself, I could keep these pounds off." You may even wonder why you can't control your cravings. You may even think it's your fault; after all, you're eating less and exercising.

There is no question that portion control and exercising are important. But as you just learned in the last chapter, our ability to lose weight also relies on a healthy liver, and most diets out there—especially the fads—don't support the liver. In fact, they encourage speedy weight loss, which itself adds to the existing burden on the liver and makes you regain the weight.

In this chapter, you are going to learn some surprising facts—ones that are causing concern among the scientific community, and are changing our ideas about what healthy weight loss really means. You will learn why most diets cause the rapid release of fats and toxins that harm the liver and keep it from doing its duties. You'll learn why these fad diets ultimately make you stop losing weight and end up at square one, and you'll find out how to prevent it, ensuring continued permanent weight loss and maximum health.

Toxic Burden on the Liver

For many people, losing weight in the early weeks of a diet is achievable. The real problem comes after that peak period, when you hit a plateau and the needle on the scale won't budge. Hunger pangs and cravings may be more frequent, but even if you resist the urge, the scale is stuck in neutral.

Some of my clients who were veteran dieters before they came to see me have said that it gets worse. They look in the mirror and think they look less youthful. They feel less vibrant. Some notice symptoms such as fatigue, mood swings, crankiness, headaches, indigestion, anxiety, and even short-term depression. It's an all-too-familiar problem for most, a situation that becomes worse when the weight begins to return.

Scientists are beginning to understand why this happens to us. We used to see body fat as collections of fat cells that just sit there and need to be dieted away as quickly as possible. But the truth is that fat stores are the body's dumping ground for harmful environmental chemicals.

Between 1970 and 1989, the Centers for Disease Control ran a program that monitored the level of toxins from human fat samples from all over the country. This program, called the National Human Adipose Tissue Survey, revealed that some of the most toxic chemicals known to humankind were stored in our fat cells.

Polychlorinated biphenyl (PCB), an industrial chemical, was found in 83 percent of all samples. Twenty toxic compounds were found in more than 76 percent of all samples. Nine harmful chemicals, including benzene, dichloro-diphenyl-trichloroethane (DDT), an insecticide, toluene, chlorobenzene, ethylbenzene, and dioxins, were found in 91 to 98 percent of all samples.

Many of these offending chemicals are organochlorines, including DDT and PCB, which were introduced in the 1950s with little knowledge of the human risks involved. These chemicals were banned in the 1970s when it was discovered that they are persistent in the environment and accumulate in the food chain, where they can harm human and animal health. One type, dioxin, is still produced as a by-product of the manufacture of PVC (polyvinyl chloride). These persistent organic chemicals, as they're called, continue to be found today in the air we breathe and in water, which is how they make their way into our food supply.

Each year, newer chemicals are introduced through the manufacture and use of consumer products such as plastics and food packaging, paint, flame retardants, cosmetics, upholstery, photocopiers and other office equipment, wallpaper, nail polish, cleaning supplies, furniture, and pesticides. Bisphenol-A, for example, is a compound that mimics estrogen and is the main component of polycarbonate, which is used to make dental sealants and hard plastic bottles. Brominated flame retardants are a widely used group of chemicals that are found in computers and mattresses.

There are an estimated eighty-two thousand chemicals being manufactured today, and an additional one thousand new chemicals are added each year. Only a fraction of these chemicals has been subjected to rigorous testing to find out if they might cause long-term health problems in humans. Many chemicals have not been scrutinized because they were created before laws were established and were exempt from evaluation. Once they are in the marketplace, they are generally not banned unless they are proven beyond a doubt to be dangerous. In contrast, the European Union adopted a proactive approach in 1992, called the precautionary principle, which allows regulators to consider potential safety risks of a chemical if there isn't conclusive evidence yet, and puts the burden on its proponents to prove that it is safe.

How do these chemicals get lodged in our fat cells to begin with? Well, once they get into our water, they wind up in food, particularly animal fat from fish, pork, beef, processed meat, milk, and cheese. They're also in the air we breathe. Thanks to newer tests that are making it possible to find ever smaller concentrations of these chemicals in people, it has already become evident to the scientific community that every one of us carries traces of synthetic chemicals in our bodies. These chemicals then get sequestered into our fat cells until they are released into the body when we shed those fat cells during a diet.

But what about the person who eats well and is generally healthy? Even "healthy" people have been found to have high levels of synthetic chemicals. For example, the *Oakland Tribune* conducted a study examining the levels of toxic chemicals in the human body. In order not to alarm readers by testing people with known exposure to these chemicals, the staff selected a family whom the project's scientific advisory board deemed low-risk—a family who ate organic food, didn't buy many new electronics or furniture, didn't have carpets, and avoided chemical cleaning products. The results, published by the *Oakland Tribune* in March 2005, were astonishing. In particular, levels of polybrominated diphenyl ether (PBDE), a flame retardant used in some upholstered furniture, carpet underlays, mattresses, computers, and other electrical equipment, were much higher than expected. Previous estimates were that people in the United States have approximately 36 parts per billion (ppb) in their blood. In the family tested, the father had 102 ppb, the mother had 138 ppb, the daughter had 490 ppb, and the son had 838 ppb. Other chemicals found were PCBs, dioxins, mercury, cadmium, and lead.

Acclaimed television journalist Bill Moyers, who won an Emmy for his work on *Trade Secrets: A Moyers Report*, a documentary about how companies worked to withhold vital information about the risks from workers, the government, and the public, had his own blood and urine tested as part of a study sponsored by Mount Sinai School of Medicine in New York. Eighty-four chemicals were found, including PCBs that had been banned for over twenty-five years.

And the thing is, the more fat we have, the more chemicals we're storing. A study published in the journal *Medicine and Science in Sports and Exercise* measured body fat and organochlorine levels in individuals with a wide range of body fat, from athletes to sedentary people of average weight to people who were overweight. The studies confirmed that across these diverse groups, the more body fat a person had, the higher the organochlorine levels in his or her body.

In another study, researchers at Laval University in Quebec, Canada, demonstrated a direct correlation between the release of organochlorine pollutants from fat stores during weight loss and the slowing of metabolic rate. The more chemicals released, the more sluggish the metabolism, more than could be attributed to dieting alone.

And a study published in the journal *Obesity Surgery* looked at organochlorine levels in people who had lost weight through diet or weight-loss surgery. After three months, people on the diet had lost 12.1 percent of their body weight and those who had surgery lost 20.9 percent of their weight. However, there was a significant increase in organochlo-rine levels. People who were classified by researchers as being obese had a 23.8 percent rise in their organochlorine levels. People who weighed more than this had a 51.8 percent increase in organochlorine levels. One year after surgery, the latter group had lost 46.3 percent of their body weight, which resulted in a 388.2 percent total increase in organochlorine levels.

So here's the first hazard of dieting: when we lose weight rapidly with the latest fad, fat stores are broken down quickly, dumping stored chem-icals into the bloodstream. This big chemical load taxes the liver (it has to process these chemicals), and it's less able to do its many weight-loss jobs. The liver can't keep up with excreting these toxins rapidly enough, so they travel to other parts of the body, such as the heart, thyroid, liver, brain, and muscles, where they slow metabolism, worsen insulin and lep-tin sensitivity, and cause cravings and fat gain in certain areas. Weight loss stops. This is also why some people develop headaches, dizziness, and fatigue while dieting.

Here's more about how this rapid release of chemicals hinders weight loss.

Released Toxins Impair Thyroid Function and Slow Metabolism

The thyroid gland, located in front of the neck, is about the same size and shape as a butterfly. The thyroid secretes two hormones, T4 (thyroxine) and T3 (triiodothyronine), which help determine the basal metabolic rate in the body, and thus influence how much weight we lose. The thyroid is also involved in the metabolism of fat, glucose, and protein, tissue growth, and proper function of the reproductive organs, nerves, heart, and bones.

Studies have found that released chemicals lower thyroid hormone lev-els and interfere with thyroid function, which results in a slower basal metabolic rate.

Symptoms of impaired thyroid function are:

- Weight gain or difficulty losing weight
- Fatigue
- Feeling cold
- Constipation, bloating

- Depression
- Forgetfulness, poor concentration
- Hair loss, dry and flaky skin
- High cholesterol
- Muscle and/or joint pain or weakness
- Heart palpitations
- Hoarseness
- Heavy menstrual periods, difficulty conceiving, miscarriage

Researchers at Laval University confirmed the connection between weight loss, organochlorine pollutants, and impaired thyroid function by tracking the levels of organochlorines, thyroid hormone (T3), and resting metabolic rate during a calorie-restricted weight-loss diet lasting fifteen weeks. They found that organochlorine levels were higher after weight loss and that the rise in these chemicals correlated with a decrease in T3 and the resting metabolic rate.

Released Toxins Cause Inflammation

Inflammation happens through different mechanisms and at different levels in the body. You may be familiar with the kind of inflammation caused by an arthritic knee, a sports injury, or a cold. But eating the wrong foods (or not eating enough of the right ones), an imbalance of bacteria in our intestines, and released toxins are some of the factors that can cause chronic low-level inflammation in the body. The more chemicals that are dumped into the bloodstream, the more our immune system is called into action. Inflammatory and anti-inflammatory substances are released into the body, which can damage our cells, organs, and arteries, and prevent sugar from getting into needy cells, promoting insulin resistance.

In addition to insulin resistance, inflammation causes cells to not properly respond to the messages of another hormone, leptin. Derived from the Greek word meaning "thin," leptin is produced by fat cells in the abdomen, and its role is to control our appetites by telling the brain how much body fat we have. Leptin works by binding to cells in the brain and blocking the release of a chemical called neuropeptide Y. The result is that you feel full and satisfied, your metabolism speeds up, and your body focuses on burning stored fat. Inflammation disrupts leptin receptors, so cells can't receive or respond to leptin's message. The result? You cannot keep your hunger or appetite in check.

Inflammation also places physical stress on the body. And as you learned in the last chapter, the stress-cortisol connection increases hunger, promotes fat storage in the abdomen, and elevates blood sugar.

Released Toxins Cause Hormonal Havoc

Many synthetic chemicals that are released into the bloodstream have an estrogen like effect in the body. Called endocrine disruptors, these chemicals mimic estrogen and disrupt our delicate hormonal balance. Although we mostly think of these hormones as related to our reproductive organs, they can have a great impact on our weight. An imbalance can affect weight gain by:

- Decreasing insulin sensitivity.
- Depositing fat in the hips, thighs, buttocks, and lower abdomen.
- Promoting cellulite formation around the hips and thighs. Excess estrogen can weaken connective tissue, the network of fibers underneath your skin. If circulation is poor, this can lead to swelling, stretching of the connective tissue, and fat protrusion, which is seen as cellulite.
- Causing water retention and bloating. Estrogen can slightly elevate aldosterone, a hormone released by our adrenal glands that makes us retain fluids and salt.
- Triggering cravings for rich, high-fat foods. Estrogen turns on a chemical called galanin, found to increase our desire for fatty foods.
- Slowing metabolism. Too much estrogen interferes with thyroid hormones.
- Causing a decline in muscle tone, which further slows metabolism. For men in particular, the increased estrogen causes a decline in free testosterone, shown to be directly related to increased fat. This also causes a decline in muscle mass, which in turn slows metabolism and elevates blood sugar.

In addition to affecting weight gain, estrogen imbalances may also be to blame for the following.

Fibroids, endometriosis
Water retention, bloating
Breast cysts or lumps

Watery eyes
Premenstrual syndrome
Menstrual periods that are heavy for more than three days
Menstrual cycle less than twenty-eight days
Varicose veins
Habitual miscarriage
Chronic sinus congestion
Insomnia
Age spots on the hands and the face
Benign prostate hypertrophy
Prostate cancer

Released Toxins Disrupt Our Blood Sugar Balance

Human and animal studies have found that persistent organochlorine pollutants are linked with the development of insulin resistance and diabetes.

- The National Health and Nutrition Examination Survey, conducted between 1999 and 2002, found that in 2,016 adults in the United States, the presence of diabetes was strongly associated with the presence of six persistent organic pollutants.
- In a study involving 196 men and 184 women, PCBs and related chemicals were significantly associated with the presence of diabetes.
- People with diabetes were found to have significantly higher levels of dioxins and PCBs.
- Exposure to an extremely low dose of bisphenol-A, a widely used chemical in plastic bottles and other food containers, has been linked with insulin resistance.

Fatty Liver

Having extra weight makes you prone to developing fatty liver. When we gain weight and accumulate excess fat, we can see it and feel it on our bodies. But we can also accumulate fat you can't see, because it's hidden in the liver. Free fatty acids (fats that are in the bloodstream) enter liver cells, where they are converted into triglycerides and stored as fat. Fat builds up in the liver.

When fat exceeds 5 percent of the liver's weight (just 0.15 pound in an average person), it's officially called fatty liver. Fatty liver is an alarmingly common condition affecting one in four people, according to a study by Johns Hopkins University School of Medicine, making it the most common liver condition in the United States. Studies have found that the greater the body mass index (BMI), the greater the degree of fatty liver. An estimated 90 percent of people who are obese or who have diabetes also have fatty liver.

As you learned earlier, conventional tests aren't sensitive enough to pick up many, if not most, causes of early liver problems, which is why most people with fatty liver don't even realize they have it. Signs of a fat-clogged liver are often subtle and nonspecific, and can include a lack of energy, indigestion, bad breath, body odor, constipation, and, of course, weight gain.

A fat-congested liver doesn't function well. It becomes less able to break down and remove fat. This is made worse by a diet rich in sweets, starchy foods, and bad fats, which can get converted into fat and add to the liver glut.

Body Mass Index Calculator

Body mass index is a measure of how much body fat we have, based on our height and weight. To find out your body mass index, or BMI:

1. Figure out your height in inches (1 foot = 12 inches). Suppose you are 5'7". Multiply 5 × 12 = 60, and add 7. Your height in inches would be 67.
2. Square that number: 67 × 67 = 4,489.
3. Take your weight, in pounds, and divide this number by the number in step 2. For example, if you are 180 pounds, divide that number by 4,489. Now multiply this number by 703. It equals 28.2, rounded off. Your BMI is 28.2.

What does this mean? The greater your BMI, the greater your chance of having fatty liver.

Underweight = below 18.5
Healthy weight = 18.5–24.9
Overweight = 25–29.9
Obese = 30 and above

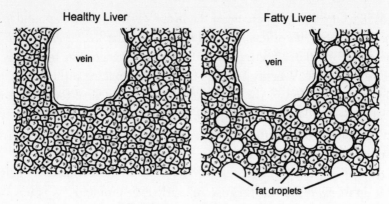

Healthy liver versus fatty liver.

This brings me to the second hazard of dieting. You have already learned about the increased toxic load of weight loss. Adding to that, many people who are overweight have fatty liver, which can compromise liver function. Then, when they go on a diet, shedded fat migrates to the liver and adds to this problem. The liver has to work extra hard to deal with the sudden burden of fat and toxins, which affects the liver's ability to do its many jobs needed for weight loss. The solution is to simultaneously support the liver while you are trying to lose weight.

Factors That Can Lead to Fatty Liver

Factors that increase the odds that you have fatty liver include the following.

Being Overweight

As I mentioned, carrying excess weight makes it more likely that you'll develop fatty liver. This is because being overweight causes changes to take place in the body. For example, free fatty acid levels are increased, which get taken up by the liver. Meanwhile, the liver has a reduced ability to use these fatty acids, so they get converted to triglycerides and stored as fat. Excess free fatty acids have also been shown to inhibit fat-burning (oxidation) in the liver.

Having Insulin Resistance or Diabetes

The excess buildup of fat in the liver is strongly associated with insulin resistance. One of insulin's actions is to drive glucose into cells, especially muscle, fat, and liver cells. It helps to think that insulin works like a lock and key. Insulin is the key that allows glucose to pass through by binding to insulin receptors (the lock) on the surface of these cells. If there is a defect in insulin receptors, insulin is less effective than it normally would be. Glucose has trouble entering cells, so the pancreas must produce more insulin to control the levels of glucose in blood. As insulin resistance progresses, even high levels of insulin are ineffective, leading to elevated blood sugar and diabetes.

The American College of Preventive Medicine calls obesity, insulin resistance, and type 2 diabetes an epidemic in the United States, where over eighty million people are insulin resistant and eighteen million have diabetes. If type 2 diabetes continues to rise following the same trends, twenty-two million people will have diabetes by 2025.

To make things worse, insulin resistance can lead to fatty liver because it changes the way sugar and fat are metabolized in the liver, muscles, and fat cells. As a result of these changes, there is an increased uptake of triglyceride fat in liver cells. This large quantity of fat comes from abdominal fat and muscles and also from our diet. The liver can't get rid of it properly, so the fat is then stored inside liver cells. Nearly everyone with fatty liver has some degree of insulin resistance, and 90 percent of people with diabetes have fatty liver.

The Inside Out Diet was developed to help prevent or correct insulin resistance. Once insulin levels are lowered and your cells are sensitive to insulin again, you can gain access to stored body fat as an energy source and also reduce fat in the liver.

Being Leptin Resistant

When we gain weight, our body fat produces more of the hormone leptin. Normally, leptin regulates weight by causing the extra pounds to be shed by suppressing appetite or increasing our metabolic rate. But with leptin resistance, cells don't receive or properly respond to leptin's signals. Not only does leptin resistance disrupt our ability to regulate weight, research indicates that leptin has an important role in determining how much liver fat we accumulate.

Eating Too Many Fatty Foods

Too much fat in the diet, especially bad fats, contributes to the problem. Elizabeth Parks, Ph.D., from the University of Minnesota, and her colleagues examined patients with fatty liver who were scheduled to have liver biopsies. They used a special marker that attached to the dietary fat they ate, so it could be distinguished from the fat that was already in the body. They also did blood tests and measured body fat. They found that all of these patients with fatty liver had high triglycerides and insulin resistance and that as much as 20 percent of the fat from the diet was found in the liver. Dr. Parks said, "The bottom line is, this is a clear indicator that if one eats too much fat, as in the film *Supersize Me*, it becomes deposited in the liver. This leads to a kind of liver toxicity that would be good to avoid."

Rapid Weight Loss Is Not the Answer

Weight loss, if it's not done properly, can overwhelm the liver with fat and further add to its burden. Because the fat stores being broken down migrate to the liver and overwhelm it, people on fad diets who lose weight quickly experience fatigue, headaches, anxiety, and general feelings of being unwell. Not only can this distract your liver from its other important duties, it can trigger inflammation in a fatty liver, a condition called nonalcoholic steatohepatitis (NASH). NASH was first termed by Jurgen Ludwig, M.D., at the Mayo Clinic after he observed that people with obesity, diabetes, and high cholesterol had a liver disease similar to alcoholic liver disease, even though they drank no alcohol. NASH can lead to scarring, liver failure, and liver cancer. Though this condition is uncommon (only about 3 percent of the general population have NASH), rapid unhealthy weight loss may actually trigger the progression to NASH in someone with fatty liver.

The Right Way to Lose Weight

By now you're probably beginning to put together the big picture of why people feel so much better—and lose weight more effectively—on my diet. By maximizing and supporting liver functioning, you can lose weight safely and permanently, without the strain, slowdowns, and symptoms of unhealthy weight loss.

What kinds of food help accomplish this? I've put together a plan, complete with delicious recipes, as part of my diet. It includes specific fruits and vegetables, in amounts that can boost liver function, decrease body fat, eliminate cravings, fight inflammation, improve insulin and leptin sensitivity, and keep you satisfied.

The meal plan includes recipes specifically designed for this diet by Sabra Ricci, a chef to celebrities and a caterer from Maui. It includes foods that give the liver the nutrients it needs to detoxify and excrete unwanted chemicals.

I've included the recipe for my Cleansing Lemon Tea, designed to help you detoxify, replenish, and rejuvenate, all at the same time. There are many other herbs and spices that help the liver and boost flavor, such as rosemary, cardamom, turmeric, and cilantro. The cilantro pesto recipe in this book is popular, and all the ingredients in it help us remove toxins, such as mercury.

You'll also enjoy the organic chicken, lamb, turkey, beef, and other high-quality sources of protein, which provide the amino acids needed by the liver to detoxify. Neither too much nor too little protein is good, and this diet gives you the optimum amount so that your liver can efficiently eliminate the stored toxins and fats. Protein, which is often lacking in detoxifying diets, is also needed to combat stress-related weight gain. That's why you'll find recipes such as Chicken Cacciatore, Maui-terranean Salad with Grilled Chicken, Thai Coconut Tempeh, and Grilled Beef Tenderloin Salad.

The colon-cleansing foods ensure that the unwanted waste that the liver discards doesn't get reabsorbed by the body. They include apples, flaxseeds, and other superfoods naturally high in soluble fiber that will bind to toxins and excess cholesterol. The diet also includes the right amount of essential fatty acids, low-glycemic foods, and other foods that decrease inflammation, restore insulin sensitivity, suppress appetite, and boost metabolism via leptin.

This diet also works at reducing toxins and inflammation produced in our bodies from food intolerances and the overgrowth of unfriendly bacteria and yeast. You'll learn how to figure out which foods, if any, you have an intolerance to and learn simple ways to get rid of unfriendly bacteria and yeast.

Although drinking too much coffee isn't recommended, you'll find out why coffee, in moderation, and green tea can actually be beneficial. You won't have to cut out coffee!

By eating the right balance of foods that help you lose weight at a steady rate, this diet maximizes your weight loss—and your health. Let's jump right in!

Misconceptions about a Detoxifying Diet

Diets that cleanse the liver are often called detox diets. Some critics call them fads and say that our bodies are built to handle toxins on their own. And while it's true that the body can detoxify itself normally, it is an overly simplistic answer, like saying we don't need antibiotics because our immune systems can fight off bacterial infections on their own. We *know* that's not true.

Part of the problem was that we had no idea just how many chemicals people really were carrying around in their bodies. Thanks to newer, more accessible tests, we can now detect very small concentrations in people's bodies, and the tests show us that our bodies cannot excrete these toxins on their own. For example, Environmental Defence Canada tested eleven people for eighty-eight potentially harmful chemicals. They found an average of forty-four chemicals, including heavy metals, and chemicals that were banned over twenty-five years ago. In collaboration with Mount Sinai School of Medicine in New York, the Environmental Working Group in Washington, D.C., released "Body Burden: The Pollution in People," a report that looked at the levels of 210 chemicals in nine people. Researchers found an average of 91 industrial compounds, pollutants, and other chemicals in the blood and urine of nine volunteers, with a total of 167 chemicals found in the group. This reinforces that our bodies are unable to deal with these chemicals without our help.

Detoxification is an ongoing process that occurs in the body. The medical community, including respected doctors such as Andrew Weil, M.D., Leo Galland, M.D., and Mark Hyman, M.D., is quickly accepting the value of eating certain foods that support this natural process.

By reviewing almost every detox diet on the shelves, I found another problem in that they are sometimes presented as restrictive, deprivation diets, meant to last only one to three weeks. These diets, paradoxically, can deplete your liver, which is your major detox organ. Some authors even promote detox diets as a way to lose weight rapidly. And detox diets usually don't allow coffee, or chicken and other animal protein; some even advise against eating any food at all. In the following chapters, I'll show you why eating many of these foods—yes, including coffee, chicken, and beef—can help you slim down safely by improving the health of your liver. And it's not going to be harsh. Quite the opposite—most people say my diet reawakens their taste buds, giving them more pleasure from food than they ever had before.

.   .   .

Now that you understand why the Inside Out Diet can help you lose weight safely and permanently, it's time to learn more about what it involves. Diet rhetoric isn't worth much if you don't put it into practice, which is why I tend to be a bit wary of any "rules" for eating in general; without any guiding principles in place, however, the risk is that you're more likely to fall prey to the next fad diet that comes by, which can wreak havoc on your physical and emotional health. The principles I lay out in the next chapters are not my personal gospel, nor do I expect you to follow them blindly. Rather, I hope that these basic food principles will make sense and provide some grounding as we move forward, helping you understand how this diet works with your body—not against it—in achieving your optimal health and weight. I will also provide you with helpful shopping tips, recipes, and other valuable information to get you started. As you are about to find out, the Inside Out Diet is not a fad, a quick fix, or a plan that you go on for one week to shed pounds quickly. It is a lifelong journey.

Part II

The Diet Code for Healthy Weight Loss

3

Give Your Tired Liver a Boost

I have everything I used to have, it's just a little lower to the ground.
—ACTRESS GYPSY ROSE LEE

Your poor liver handles much of the burden of detoxification, so to keep the process running smoothly when faced with the increased chemical burden of weight loss, you need to provide it with the protein, vitamins, minerals, and nutrients it needs to properly do its job.

Make "Whey" for a Liver-Healthy Food

Chances are, you may have not even thought of, let alone tried, this by-product of cheese-making made famous by little Miss Muffet and her curds-and-whey diet. Whey, the watery part of milk that separates from the solid curds, has become popular as a protein powder, and with good reason. Whey contains all the essential amino acids (the ones we must obtain through our diet), making it a complete protein. It is particularly rich in cysteine, the amino acid that is needed to make glutathione, one of the most potent antioxidants and detoxifiers in the body.

Glutathione is a protein made in the body from three amino acids: cysteine, glycine, and glutamic acid. Although it's used in every cell in the body, it's found in highest concentrations in the liver. Glutathione is particularly good at seeking and eliminating the toxic substances released by fat cells during weight loss, such as PCBs and other industrial chemicals. In fact, over 60 percent of the toxins that go to the liver are detoxified by glutathione. So having adequate glutathione is essential for continued weight loss, and you need to make sure you eat foods that will replenish it.

Glutathione also functions as an antioxidant, fighting the free radicals generated during weight loss. That's why glutathione is an especially important part of this diet. Glutathione gets used up faster when we lose weight. Other contributors to this loss are stress, liver disease, poor diet, alcohol, diabetes, cigarette smoking, pollution, chemicals, painkillers, and infection. Glutathione also protects the immune system and recycles vitamins E and C.

Whey also has these additional benefits for weight and health:

- Decreases body fat by suppressing fatty-acid synthesis
- Improves insulin sensitivity
- Decreases postmeal spikes in blood sugar
- Promotes weight loss
- Increases levels of serotonin, which helps curb cravings for sweet and starchy foods
- Improves liver function and protects cells against inflammation, free radicals, and oxidative stress
- Contains branched-chain amino acids, which are important for lean muscle growth and the repair of body tissues
- Conserves vitamin E in the body
- Protects arteries from damage
- Increases taurine, an amino acid that prevents gallstone formation, reduces triglycerides, and allows cholesterol to be cleared from the body. Studies have found that it also lowers body weight and suppresses the sympathetic nervous system.

How to Do It: Each day, have one scoop of whey protein powder. You can find it in health food stores and on the shelves in the vitamin section of many supermarkets. Most containers come with a scoop inside. Read the label to find out how much protein is in each scoop. Look for one with 10 to 24 grams of protein per scoop. Be sure to look for whey protein isolate (not the concentrate), which is over 90 percent whey protein and has very little lactose and fat, and if you can, try to find one that is organic.

Whey protein comes in vanilla, chocolate, and strawberry, but flavored whey tends to have artificial colors and sweeteners, so check the label before buying.

Whey protein mixes well into smoothies and adds a nice thickness and a rich, creamy taste. If you don't like smoothies, try mixing whey protein into yogurt and topping it with fresh berries, or mixing it into milk to have with breakfast cereal.

Eat More Cruciferous Vegetables

There are plenty of great reasons to include more cruciferous veggies like broccoli and cauliflower in your diet. This family of vegetables is called the crucifers, because of the flowers that often bloom in the shape of a cross. They contain a variety of healthy compounds, including sulforaphane, first discovered by Dr. Paul Talalay, M.D., at Johns Hopkins University. Talalay identified this particular compound in broccoli, cabbage, watercress, and other cruciferous vegetables as having the greatest ability to produce detoxifying enzymes. He later found that broccoli sprouts, which look like alfalfa sprouts but are not as thready, have ten to one hundred times more sulforaphane than broccoli does.

Cruciferous vegetables include the following:

Arugula	Brussels sprouts	Mustard greens
Bok choy	Cabbage	Rutabaga
Broccoli	Cauliflower	Swiss chard
Broccolini	Chinese cabbage	Turnip greens
Broccoli rabe	Collard greens	Turnips
Broccoli sprouts	Kale	Watercress

Sulforaphane, an antioxidant, speeds up the detoxification of many potentially harmful chemicals, enhances glutathione production, and is believed to prevent cancer and suppress tumor growth.

Another compound in crucifers called indole-3-carbinol has been found to increase the detoxification of estrogen in the liver by as much as 50 percent. This makes it extremely beneficial during weight loss, when the liver is inundated with estrogenlike chemicals from fat stores. Indole-3-carbinol is also believed to fight cancer, especially breast and prostate cancer.

How to Do It: Aim for at least two servings of cruciferous vegetables per day (1 serving = $\frac{1}{2}$ cup cooked, 1 cup raw, or $\frac{1}{4}$ cup broccoli sprouts). One way is to add arugula to your salad. While most of us think of arugula as an alternative to lettuce, it's actually a cruciferous vegetable and contains more vitamin C and calcium than any other salad green, along with folic acid and other vitamins and minerals. If you find arugula's pungent, peppery bite to be a bit overwhelming, look for baby arugula, which is less peppery and hot, or try mixing it with other salad greens to soften the taste. Arugula salads taste good with dressings made with lemon juice, balsamic vinegar, extra-virgin olive oil, or hazelnut oil.

Another option is cauliflower, one of the few cruciferous vegetables (along with turnips) that can be used as a substitute for starchy foods. Try chopping it finely in the food processor to simulate the texture of rice, or mashing it—a healthier option as it contains about a third of the calories of potatoes. Try the delicious Chicken Stir-Fry over "Rice" recipe in this book, which uses cauliflower instead of rice. My favorite way to eat cauliflower is as a snack. I chop it into bite-size pieces, toss it with extra-virgin olive oil and a bit of sea salt, and roast it in the oven until it's lightly browned. You can add cumin, cayenne, or other spices for added flavor.

Have no more than one serving of *raw* cruciferous vegetables a day, because large quantities can impair thyroid function. Any cooking, whether it's steaming, boiling, baking, roasting, grilling, or microwaving, deactivates the unwanted thyroid-impairing compounds.

Eat in Color

The pigment of each fruit and vegetable offers more than aesthetic appeal. We can actually categorize a plant's particular nutritional value based on its color, which is caused by phytonutrients or plant nutrients. Each pigment packs a powerful punch in terms of your body's ability to lose weight.

The Purple Protectors (Purple or Red in Color)

This group contains anthocyanins (pronounced an-tho-*sigh*-uh-nins), water-soluble antioxidants that reduce the risk of cancer, heart disease, diabetes, and allergies, and prevent DNA damage, inflammation, and premature aging. A vital part of the diet, this group has the following specific benefits:

- Supports the production of adiponectin, a hormone that suppresses appetite and helps turn body fat into energy
- Has natural anti-inflammatory properties that improve insulin and leptin sensitivity
- Strengthens blood vessels and capillaries, reducing varicose veins and cellulite formation
- Helps prevent obesity
- Is high in fiber (especially raspberries)
- Reduces the breakdown of collagen by inflammatory chemicals, which helps prevent skin aging
- Enhances glutathione production, improving liver function and detoxification

Fruits and vegetables in this group include:

Beets	Cranberries	Raspberries
Blackberries	Eggplant	Red apples
Black currants	Plums	Strawberries
Blueberries	Pomegranates	
Cherries	Purple cabbage	

Beets are loaded with betaine, a liver-protecting antioxidant that has been found to help the liver process fats and prevent fat from accumulating in the liver. In one study, betaine supplements significantly improved liver enzymes and decreased fat deposits in the liver. Animal studies also show that betaine can improve liver function and protect against chemical damage to the liver.

Blueberries are one of the highest in antioxidants of any fruit or vegetable. They contain the phytochemical anthocyanidins and are rich in pectin, the fiber that binds to toxins and also helps lower cholesterol. Blueberries also have a compound similar to cranberries, called epicatechin, and can be used to prevent urinary tract infections.

Raspberries, strawberries, and pomegranates contain ellagic acid, a compound that has been found to protect against liver damage, enhance glutathione, neutralize toxins, and reduce the weight effects of endocrine-disruptors.

Raspberries are particularly good for you. Japanese researchers recently isolated a compound in raspberries that has unique weight-loss effects. They gave animals a high-fat diet for ten weeks and found that supplementing the diet with the raspberry compound reduced abdominal fat, triglycerides, total body fat, and overall weight, and improved their ability to burn fat.

How to Do It: Each day, eat at least one serving (1 serving = ¾ cup) of the purple protectors, whether it's adding a handful of fresh or frozen berries to your breakfast, enjoying a raspberry or blueberry smoothie or pomegranate juice during the day, or having berries topped with a tablespoon of sliced almonds for a simple but delicious dessert!

Try having beets with dinner. Beets can be boiled, pureed, roasted, grilled, or pickled. Boil them unpeeled and leave at least an inch of the green stem so the color doesn't bleed. Raw beets can be grated into salads or juiced with other vegetables. If you don't have time to cook them, look for canned beets at the grocery store. Avoid jarred beets, which usually come with added sugar. Beets have an earthy sweetness that is best complemented in salads by vinaigrette with lemon, apple cider vinegar, or balsamic vinegar, and bold flavors such as arugula, olives, and feta cheese.

If you are pressed for time, try unsweetened pomegranate juice, which has a deep red color and a tart taste. Blueberry juice is another option. You can drink the juice, or try mixing ¼ cup of pomegranate juice with a single serving of nonfat organic vanilla yogurt in a cup for a quick smoothie. Although you lose the fiber by drinking rather than eating these fruits, you'll still enjoy the other health benefits of eating these purple protectors.

The Extraordinary Oranges (Yellow, Orange, or Green in Color)

This is the largest group, containing fat-soluble phytonutrients called carotenoids (pronounced car-*ott*-eh-noyds). As the name implies, these plant pigments give carrots their orange color. This group contains vegetables and fruits ranging from yellow to green to orange because the green-pigmented chlorophyll that gives plants their characteristic green color can overshadow the orange pigment in certain foods.

Beta-carotene is the best known carotenoid, but this group also includes other carotenoids such as lutein (pronounced *loo*-teen), lycopene, alpha-carotene, and foods rich in vitamin C and the related bioflavonoids. The following vegetables and fruits contain carotenoids:

Vegetables

Bell peppers	Squash	
Carrots	Sweet	
Green beans	potatoes	
Leafy greens	Tomatoes	
Lettuce	Zucchini	
Peas, green		
Peppers		
Pumpkin		
Spinach		

Fruit

Apricots	Nectarines
Cantaloupes	Oranges
Clementines	Passionfruit
Grapefruit,	Peaches
pink	Pears
Guava	Persimmons
Honeydew	Tangerines
Kiwi	Watermelon
Lemons	

The extraordinary oranges carry out a variety of important functions needed for weight loss.

- They protect our cell membranes (which are composed of more than 30 percent fat) and other tissues from toxin damage during weight loss.
- They improve the sensitivity of insulin.
- In particular, lycopene, a carotenoid found in tomatoes, reduces the risk of cardiovascular disease.

The orange group also contains foods high in vitamin C, which is important during weight loss for the following reasons:

- Aids in the formation of the appetite-quashing neurotransmitters serotonin and dopamine
- Helps prevent stress-related weight gain in the abdomen
- Boosts glutathione levels and is involved in deactivating toxins
- Reduces inflammation by influencing histamine release and degradation
- Lowers the amount of cholesterol in bile by converting cholesterol to bile acids, making bile less likely to clump together and form stones (studies have linked vitamin C deficiency to gallstone formation)

Some of the foods that are higher in vitamin C include citrus, watermelon, red bell peppers, cantaloupe, and kiwi. But my top pick for vitamin C is guava. Guava, a yellowish green tropical fruit, though harder to find in the grocery store than other fruits, rates high in vitamin C. One guava has approximately 165 mg and only 46 calories, compared to an orange, which has 75 mg of vitamin C and 60 calories. Guava is also one of the highest in fiber and contains vitamin E. Look for guava in Asian grocery stores and some supermarkets. Avoid guava juice, which is sweetened.

How to Do It: Include at least two servings (½ cup each) of the extraordinary oranges every day. Try adding diced bell peppers or frozen chopped spinach to a breakfast omelet, packing grape or cherry tomatoes to have with lunch, or microwaving frozen peas, green beans, or a small sweet potato to have with your dinner instead of a white potato. If you usually have a salad, try grating raw carrots into the salad and substituting spinach instead of lettuce.

Antioxidant All-Stars

Researchers at the Agricultural Research Service's Human Research Center on Aging at Tufts University have identified the fruits and vegetables that have the highest naturally occurring antioxidants, identified by an analysis called the ORAC, short for oxygen radical absorbance capacity. These fruits and vegetables protect cells from oxidative damage. Note that although the two highest scoring fruits are prunes and raisins, they are also higher in sugar.

Top Antioxidant Foods

Fruit	ORAC Units per 100 Grams (about 3½ ounces)	Vegetables	ORAC Units per 100 Grams (about 3½ ounces)
Prunes	5,770	Garlic	1,940
Raisins	2,830	Kale	1,770
Blueberries	2,400	Spinach	1,260
Blackberries	2,036	Brussels sprouts	980
Strawberries	1,540	Broccoli florets	890
Raspberries	1,220	Beets	840
Plums	949	Bell pepper, red	710
Oranges	750	Onion	450
Grapes, red	739	Corn	400
Cherries	670	Eggplant	390
Kiwi	602		
Grapefruit, pink	483		

The Right Whites (White or Light Green in Color)

If you are one of the many people who enjoy cooking with garlic and onions, including more of these foods in your diet should be easy. The active phytonutrient in this family, called allicin, has been shown to lower cholesterol and blood pressure, prevent cancer, and enhance overall health. Here are just a few of the weight-loss and health benefits of this flavorful group:

- Lowers total cholesterol, increases healthy HDL cholesterol, and prevents the harmful oxidation of LDL cholesterol
- Reduces high blood pressure and prevents clot formation
- Improves sensitivity of cells to insulin and leptin
- Destroys harmful bacteria, yeast, and fungi in the intestines
- Improves detoxification by increasing the production of glutathione, allowing for the effective elimination of toxins and carcinogenic substances

Foods in this group are:

| Chives | Garlic | Onions | Shallots |
| Endives | Leeks | Scallions | |

How to Do It: Aim for at least one serving of the right whites each day (1 serving = ¼ cup or 1 clove of garlic). Onions, garlic, shallots, chives, and scallions enhance the flavor of many foods. If the thought of eating raw garlic makes you cringe, start with one clove, which still gives you a good amount of allicin (at least 10 mg) but usually doesn't result in a detectable garlic odor. It should be crushed or chopped and added to food to release the allicin, rather than eaten whole.

Get Picky about Protein

Including some animal protein in your diet can greatly improve the health of the liver. This may be contrary to what you've read elsewhere, but protein helps to curb hunger, and animal protein has these additional fat-burning and detoxifying nutrients:

- The nutrient carnitine helps burn fat for fuel by carrying it to the energy-producing portion of the cell. Preliminary studies show that carnitine can reduce fat deposits in the liver and protect the heart by increasing good HDL cholesterol and lowering triglycerides. Carnitine is found in beef and lamb.

- The sulfur-containing amino acids methionine and cysteine are two of the most important nutrients for detoxification. Legumes and nuts have about half as much of these amino acids as animal protein, and other plant foods have only 10 to 20 percent compared with an equivalent amount of animal protein.

And finally, if you are trying to lose weight, eliminating animal protein can make you shed pounds too quickly, flooding the body with toxins that can't be properly eliminated because you don't have enough of the necessary amino acids to support this process.

What's most important is choosing lean protein sources with the least contamination. Here are my top picks:

- *Organic poultry.* Besides containing fewer chemicals, many people say that organic chicken is far better tasting than nonorganic. In order to make fewer trips to the health food grocery, try buying larger quantities and freezing them. You can also alternate between boneless and bone-in, which costs less. For breakfast, there are organic chicken breakfast links (such as Han's and Applegate Farms) and turkey bacon (Wellshire Farms) that are made without the preservatives nitrite or nitrate. The animals are raised without antibiotics, and the meat is lower in sodium.

  Tip: If you don't have time to cook, try picking up a plain organic rotisserie chicken and serving the sliced meat (without the skin) over brown rice and a tomato-arugula salad. The leftovers make for a tasty lunch the next day.

- *Grass-fed beef.* Beef from cows that have been raised on a grass-based diet, which is more consistent with their natural habitat, contains more omega-3 fatty acids and less saturated fats than regular beef. These health benefits are lost when animals are fed grains such as corn, wheat, barley, and oats, which is the norm today because grains are cheap and readily available.

- *Lamb.* Lamb is one of the best sources of carnitine. Although lamb generally isn't considered one of the leanest meats, certain cuts, such as loin chops or leg shank, are lower in fat than other cuts of lamb. Any visible fat should be trimmed.

- *Omega-3 eggs.* Egg whites provide high-quality protein and also contain sulfur, which is needed for liver detoxification and proper bile flow. In step 1 of the Inside Out Diet, try liquid egg whites (e.g., Eggology), which are usually in the refrigerated section of the grocery store beside whole eggs. Adding ⅛ of a teaspoon of the mild-tasting spice turmeric to two egg whites gives them a natural yellow color that makes it look like you're eating the whole egg.

   Whole eggs, in moderation, do not appear to raise cholesterol. In a randomized controlled study, healthy adults ate either two eggs or oatmeal a day for six weeks. After the six weeks, the people who ate eggs didn't have higher cholesterol. The researchers stated that "dietary cholesterol may be less detrimental to cardiovascular health than previously thought." If you do eat eggs, however, I suggest poaching, boiling, or frying them on low heat, keeping the yolk intact, and eating scrambled eggs no more than twice a week. Otherwise, oxidized cholesterol may form, which appears to lead to atherosclerosis and heart disease. The egg yolks are also high in an inflammation-promoting substance called arachidonic acid, which is why whole eggs are limited to six or less a week in step 2.

   Choose eggs that are labeled "omega-3" or high in "DHA," a type of omega-3 fatty acid. Regular chickens are now routinely fed diets high in omega-6 oils, which means their eggs contain less of the healthy omega-3 fatty acids and more omega-6. A study published in the *New England Journal of Medicine* found that free-range eggs contain nearly twenty times more omega-3 fats than the eggs of standard corn-fed chickens.

   Omega-3 eggs usually come from chickens that have been fed algae or flaxseeds. One omega-3 egg is approximately equivalent to one 3-ounce serving of salmon in terms of omega-3 content.

Eat Certain Fish in Moderation

Fish and seafood are among the most contaminated foods in our diet. In general, certain species of fish and seafood are less contaminated than others (although there is also a lot of variation, depending on how polluted the surrounding water is). Although there are many benefits to eating fish and seafood and they taste good, I don't suggest you eat them for their omega fatty acids. The higher-fat, cold-water fish that are the best sources of omega fatty acids are usually the most contaminated with chemicals.

Omega fatty acid supplements, which I'll tell you about later, are a great alternative. They are capsules of the extracted fish oil that have had the mercury, PCBs, and other chemicals removed.

Wild Salmon

Many chemicals are turning up in areas we used to consider to be pristine, such as the Arctic, where much wild salmon originates. Marla Cone, environmental reporter for the *Los Angeles Times*, discusses in her book *Silent Snow: The Slow Poisoning of the Arctic*, how chemicals are carried by water and air to the Arctic. Because there is less soil and vegetation there to absorb these environmental pollutants, they're more likely to end up in humans, animals, and fish living there. A recent survey of the Arctic found that new chemicals are turning up in humans in increasing levels. The problem is serious enough that it has prompted international action.

So, although most wild salmon is less contaminated than farmed salmon, we should still be mindful of how much we are eating. For example, a study published in the journal *Science* tested for organochlorines in two metric tons of farmed and wild salmon from around the world. The researchers concluded that consumption of wild Alaskan salmon, in order to meet the U.S. Enviromental Protection Agency (EPA) cumulative risk assessment, should be limited to four servings a month or less.

Now you may be thinking, "Sure, but how can I possibly afford wild salmon?" You can afford it if you buy canned Alaskan salmon. Because this wonderful source of salmon is in a remote area and large amounts of fish are caught in a relatively short time, over 90 percent of Alaskan salmon are canned or frozen. That's right, canned salmon are typically wild Alaskan salmon. According to the Alaska Seafood Marketing Institute, the two most commonly canned Alaska salmon are sockeye (also known as "red" salmon) and pink salmon. Pink salmon is one of the least contaminated of all wild salmon. It's also the most abundant and therefore the least expensive, making up more than half of the U.S. commercial wild salmon catch.

Here are some of the varieties of wild salmon:

- *Pink salmon.* The smallest and youngest of the salmon. Therefore, it is the least contaminated and the least expensive. It comes from marine fisheries, not fish farms, and contains less oil than sockeye but more than chum. A three-and-a-half ounce serving of canned salmon will still give you one gram of omega-3s. It is my top pick.

- *Sockeye salmon.* Also called red salmon. It is found fresh, frozen, and canned and is an excellent choice for fresh salmon.

- *Chum.* The least contaminated of all wild salmon. More than 85 percent are from Alaska, which has the second largest chum fishery in the world, after Japan. It also has the lowest oil content of wild salmon. I find the taste variable and prefer pink salmon.

- *Coho.* Also called silver salmon. It accounts for less than 10 percent of the wild salmon caught in the United States. The quality is considered much higher than chum, and it's less expensive than sockeye or chinook.

Small, Nonpredatory Fish and Seafood

Nonpredatory fish don't feed on other fish, so they accumulate fewer chemicals. Seafood in this category are anchovy, herring, sardines, and tilapia.

Fish and Seafood to Avoid

Farmed Salmon

Farmed salmon production has risen by more than 400 percent in the last decade, and yet it's believed to be the most PCB-contaminated protein source in our food supply. These fish have significantly higher levels of PCBs, dioxin, and other chemical contaminants. They are sometimes fed fish meal from larger and more contaminated fish.

Also, because of a shortage of marine resources, vegetable oils such as corn oil are increasingly being used in fish farms as feed. The problem is that salmon convert much of the vegetable oil to arachidonic acid, which ends up in their fat. In humans, arachidonic acid is linked to inflammation and insulin resistance, arthritis, heart disease, obesity, and other diseases. The Women's Healthy Eating and Living Study of 179 women found that arachidonic acid was linked to damage to our genetic material.

Just consider the numbers: according to the United States Department of Agriculture (USDA), a 4-ounce piece of wild salmon has 267 milligrams of arachidonic acid, whereas the same-size piece of farmed salmon has 1,152 milligrams of arachidonic acid. That's four times the amount in wild salmon, and that's bad!

Wild Chinook Salmon

Also called king salmon, wild chinook salmon is the largest of the salmon and also the most contaminated, even in the wild. Chinook is also the most expensive of the salmon and is often found in high-end restaurants.

Predatory Fish

Predatory fish are higher on the food chain, so they accumulate all the chemicals in the fish they eat. They include bass, king mackerel, shark, swordfish, tilefish, tuna, and walleye.

Bottom-Feeding Fish and Seafood

Bottom-feeders reside at the bottom of lakes, seas, and oceans, which puts them amid the sediments where mercury, dioxins, and other chemicals settle. They include oysters, mussels, lobster, shrimp, and crab.

How to Do It: Aim for one to two servings of high-quality, lean protein a day (1 serving = 3 ounces of meat or 4 ounces of fish for women and 4 ounces of meat or 5 ounces of fish for men). Replace unhealthy fish and meat with the healthier options I've discussed. Instead of shellfish and farmed salmon, choose wild salmon (especially canned wild Alaskan pink salmon), anchovies, sardines, and other fish such as tilapia, but eat them no more than once a week.

Try ordering bone-in poultry, or freezing larger orders of poultry and meat, which can cut your grocery bill. Check the resources section in the back of this book for more information on where to find organic meat in your area. If you don't eat meat, eat more oats, whole eggs, and whey, which naturally have more of the liver-friendly amino acids methionine and cysteine.

Cook with Detoxifying Herbs and Spices

Herbs and spices are an important part of the Inside Out Diet, because of their potent detoxifying, weight-loss, and anti-inflammatory effects. Not only that, they enhance the taste of food. A little pinch goes a long way.

- *Cardamom.* A spice that originated in India, cardamom is a liver protector that also contains volatile oils that aid digestion and relieve gas. Use it to enhance the flavor of sweet potatoes, chicken, lentils, squash, brown rice, or peas, or try adding ⅛ teaspoon to your coffeemaker for a flavor boost.

- *Cayenne.* Traditionally known as a blood purifier that also helps to elim- inate fluids, cayenne has been found to enhance circulation (which helps us detoxify), reduce cholesterol and triglycerides, prevent free- radical damage in the liver, and boost metabolism.

- *Cilantro (Coriander leaves).* Cilantro mobilizes stored mercury, alu- minum, tin, and lead so they can be excreted. It goes well with lentils, tomatoes, salsa, chicken, rice, and salads.

- *Cumin.* Cumin is an antioxidant, anti-inflammatory, and liver healer that raises glutathione levels, boosts circulation, and improves the flow of bile. Try it with cabbage, beans, curry, peas, or chicken.

- *Dill.* Dill is particularly good at protecting us against chemicals such as those in cigarette smoke and barbecued foods. The feathery leaves pair well with beets, yogurt sauces, cucumbers, salmon, and other fish.

- *Parsley.* Parsley is an ideal herb for weight loss. It is high in vitamin C, beta-carotene, chlorophyll, and folic acid, which are all needed for detoxification. Parsley also boosts glutathione, normalizes blood sugar, and protects against liver dysfunction caused by insulin resistance. Chopped parsley can be added to any salad or even made into a pesto. The two popular types are curly parsley and Italian or flat-leaf parsley. Choose Italian parsley, which isn't as bitter and has a better flavor than curly.

- *Peppermint.* Peppermint dissolves gallstones, relieves digestive spasms to decrease gas, and improves digestion. This clean-tasting herb is best as an herbal tea. The chopped fresh herb can also be added as a gar- nish for fruit.

- *Rosemary.* The essential oils in rosemary are known to be energizing. Rosemary helps to improve circulation, relieves stress-related exhaus- tion, and protects the liver against damage caused by certain medica- tions. It tastes great with beans, sardines, roasted vegetables, anchovies, and chicken.

- *Thyme.* A member of the mint family and one of the most popular herbs, thyme is a delicious complement to bean, vegetable, fish, and egg dishes. In animal studies, thyme has been found to protect and improve the amount of omega fatty acids in cell membranes.

- *Turmeric.* Best known as the pigment that makes curry powder yellow, turmeric has been used for thousands of years in ayurvedic medicine to protect the liver. It is also used to relieve digestive problems such as discomfort, bloating, and gas. Turmeric contains curcumin, a bioflavonoid in the pigment that has been found to protect the liver, help the liver clear toxic chemicals, prevent fat deposits in the liver, fight inflammation, scavenge free radicals, and protect DNA. Try adding ⅛ teaspoon of turmeric powder to two egg whites for a natural yellow color, or adding it to soup.

- *Other herbs and spices to use.* These include basil, caraway, cloves, chile, horseradish, and oregano. Try cooking with these spices, which naturally increase the sweetness of food without the calories: cinnamon, vanilla, allspice, ginger, fenugreek, and nutmeg.

How to Do It: Find new ways to include detoxifying herbs and spices with your daily meals.

Include Liver-Friendly Nutrients in Your Diet

A daily multivitamin ensures that you are getting the nutritional support your liver needs to do its job and keeps your metabolism humming along. One of the most important vitamins is folic acid, and it is also the most common vitamin deficiency in the world. A deficiency of folic acid can lead to the buildup of a harmful compound called homocysteine.

Homocysteine is produced during the metabolism of the essential amino acid methionine. Methionine donates part of itself, the methyl group, so that the body can detoxify harmful substances, create brain chemicals, and repair damaged cells. What remains is homocysteine, a toxic by-product. Homocysteine either needs to be converted back to methionine or used to create cysteine, which is essential for glutathione production, and taurine, which is needed for smooth bile. Abnormally high levels of homocysteine in the blood are a sign that there is a breakdown in this process. Among its far-reaching negative health effects are the following:

- Harms the liver by increasing free radical damage and impairing detoxification. It may also promote liver fibrosis (scarring). High blood levels of homocysteine are prevalent in people with liver disease.
- Is an independent risk factor for heart disease when blood levels are high. Measuring homocysteine is especially useful in people who

may not have high blood pressure or other risk factors, yet have a family history of heart disease.

- Raises LDL cholesterol.

High homocysteine levels have also been linked to depression, osteoporosis, Alzheimer's disease, Parkinson's disease, chronic fatigue syndrome, fibromyalgia, eye conditions, erectile dysfunction, diabetes, ulcerative colitis, and lupus.

Folic acid is involved in every bodily function that requires cell division. It generates red blood cells, helps wounds to heal, builds muscle, and produces brain and nervous-system chemicals. There are often few or no obvious symptoms of moderate folic acid deficiency, which makes it difficult to detect.

Folic acid is the most common deficiency in the world due to the high consumption of animal foods and the low intake of vegetables and legumes. Folic acid is found in high concentrations in spinach, kale, and other cruciferous vegetables, as well as in beans and whole grains.

Vitamins B12 and B6 are important when increased levels of toxic chemicals are present (such as during weight loss). They are needed for the formation of the liver nutrients cysteine and methionine, which protect the liver and promote the elimination of chemicals.

Vitamin E also plays a beneficial role in liver health during weight loss because people with low levels of vitamin E may not be able to decrease liver fat through diet alone.

Essential minerals for detoxification include selenium and zinc.

How to Do It: Take a multivitamin every day. It should contain all of the above vitamins and minerals and meet these liver-friendly guidelines:

- It doesn't have iron, unless you are a premenopausal or pregnant woman or have iron-deficiency anemia.
- It doesn't have artificial colors.
- Vitamin A from "retinol," "retinyl palmitate," or "retinyl acetate" should not exceed 5,000 IU per day. People with some liver diseases may need even less.

For additional tips and recommendations on multivitamins, visit the Inside Out Diet Web site at www.iodiet.com.

4

Cleanse Your Colon

I come from a family where gravy is considered a beverage.
—HUMORIST ERMA BOMBECK

The cholesterol, toxins, and other waste that bile dumps into the colon need something to stick to (fiber), or they just get reabsorbed back into the body, defeating the whole purpose of liver function. Fiber and water keep bowel movements regular. Constipation, bad breath, body odor, bulging abdomen, and bloating are signs of a poorly functioning colon.

Eat Flaxseeds

Flaxseeds are shiny, reddish-brown or golden seeds that are the size of sesame seeds. They provide high amounts of soluble and insoluble fiber, contain cancer-fighting compounds called lignans, are a source of the healthy fat alpha-linoleic acid, and are relatively inexpensive.

Flaxseeds are found in health food stores and some supermarkets. They have been used by European bakers for many years and are now found in many breads, chips, and other foods. I really enjoy the taste of ground flaxseeds and sprinkle them on vegetables, brown rice, and many other dishes. You can also do the same with the recipes in this book. The added fiber slows the movement of glucose into the blood, which means there is no rapid surge or drop in blood sugar and you stay full longer. I prefer the taste of flaxseeds to psyllium husks, another source of fiber, and think you will, too. Flaxseeds should be stored in an airtight jar in the fridge.

The following are some of flaxseed's flab-fighting benefits:

- Curbs hunger.
- Prevents spikes in blood sugar.
- Binds with estrogen receptors, blocking weight gain due to hormone-disrupting chemicals.
- Lowers cholesterol by binding bile acids and preventing reabsorption into the blood. Also lowers triglycerides.
- Prevents stagnation of bile and reduces gallstone formation.
- Promotes regular bowel movements and speeds the elimination of toxins and other unwanted substances. The insoluble fiber in flaxseeds is a natural laxative.
- Contains lignans, which appear to have a protective effect in breast and prostate cancers.

You can buy whole flaxseeds and grind them yourself, or buy them already ground in vacuum-sealed bags. For convenience, I usually buy ground flaxseeds.

Because flaxseeds contain cyanogenic glycosides, overconsumption (more than 3–4 tablespoons a day) can suppress the thyroid's ability to take up sufficient iodine, which can lead to goiter. I suggest toasting flaxseeds at 250 degrees for 15 minutes to deactivate the glycosides if you eat more than 3 tablespoons a day.

How to Do It: Include 1 to 2 tablespoons of ground flaxseeds in your diet each day. Try mixing ground flaxseeds into brown rice, quinoa, or vegetables; sprinkling it on oatmeal or breakfast cereal; or adding it to a smoothie. You can also try making the flaxseed crackers in the recipe section of this book.

Choose Toxin-Binding Foods

Foods that are high in a particular type of fiber, called soluble fiber, are especially good at getting rid of excess cholesterol, toxins, and unwanted waste. Soluble fiber has the following benefits:

- Acts like a sponge that soaks up toxins and moves them through the intestines faster
- Slows the absorption of sugar into the bloodstream, allowing you to maintain stable blood sugar and control your appetite
- Soaks up fat and slows fat absorption in the intestines
- Lowers elevated cholesterol by binding with bile acids in the intestines
- Curbs hunger, because fiber stays in the stomach longer and absorbs water, making you feel full

The National Cholesterol Education Program advises eating as much as 10 to 25 milligrams of soluble fiber a day, but recent studies suggest most of us only get about 3 to 4 grams of soluble fiber a day in our diet. Without it, we can't properly remove toxins and lose weight.

How to Do It: Each day, have a minimum of one serving of colon-cleansing foods: apples (1 medium or ½ cup applesauce), pears (1 medium), grapefruit (1 small), beans or legumes (½ cup cooked), oats (½ cup cooked), artichokes (1 large or ½ cup artichoke hearts), shirataki noodles (½ cup), carob powder (¼ cup), or fiber powder (1 serving glucomannan, acacia, guar gum, psyllium, or methylcellulose powders with water). Make sure you drink enough water because fiber absorbs water. Otherwise, fiber can cause constipation. If you experience bloating or gas with fiber powder, cut back on the amount or try another brand.

Apples are a great choice because they contain calcium d-glucarate, which enhances the elimination of estrogenic compounds. They are also high in insoluble fiber and the soluble fiber pectin. Although unpeeled apples are best, peeled apples retain the pectin, so you can also try individual containers of unsweetened applesauce for variety. Look for the chunky kind.

Pears contain even more pectin than apples, helping bind with toxins in the intestines and curb hunger. Researchers from the State University of Rio de Janeiro studied the impact of apples and pears on weight loss. They found that overweight women who ate 300 grams of apples or pears—the equivalent of three small fruits—a day lost more weight on a low-calorie plan than women who didn't add apples and pears to their diet. In addition, the women who ate these fruits ate fewer calories overall.

Oats are an excellent source of soluble fiber. They contain twice the protein of brown rice and also have selenium, a mineral needed for detoxification. I recommend that you try old-fashioned rolled oats, where the whole grain is rolled and is left intact. They take about five minutes to cook. Most people prefer the taste to quick-cooking or instant oats. Old-fashioned oats don't raise blood sugar as much as instant or quick-cooking oats, so they will help you feel full for a longer time.

Steel-cut oats, also called Irish oatmeal or Scotch oats, are another healthy choice. They have a dense, chewy texture. Because they haven't been pressed flat with steel rollers, they take longer to cook than rolled oats.

Artichokes are extremely popular in Europe, not just as a food but as a liver and digestive tonic that's beneficial during weight loss. The artichoke plant is a tall thistlelike plant, and the part we eat is the unopened flower bud. The active compounds are called caffeoylquinic acids, or cynarin, which are found in highest concentration in the leaves but are also found in the artichoke heart. These liver-friendly compounds prevent the build up of fat and toxins in the liver, reduce gallstone formation during weight loss, promote the growth of beneficial bacteria in the intestines, and act as a gentle laxative by increasing bile secretion.

Artichokes contain inulin, which is a type of carbohydrate called fructan. Inulin is only slightly digested in the small intestine and has been shown to decrease ghrelin, the hormone produced by the stomach that makes you want to eat, and modulate the production of other chemicals involved in appetite regulation. Inulin has also been found to reduce the formation of fat in the liver.

Although fresh is best, health food stores and some supermarkets carry frozen artichoke hearts, which are a convenient alternative. If you're not able to find them, look for jarred artichoke hearts packed in water. Avoid oil-packed artichokes. *Caution*: Artichoke extracts shouldn't be used by people with gallstones or bile duct occlusion.

Beans and legumes are another rich source of soluble fiber. To save time, try red lentils, which cook faster than any other bean or legume and don't require soaking. Canned beans and legumes can also be used, but they should be rinsed thoroughly to remove the added salt.

Carob powder comes from the pods of the carob tree and is a member of the legume (pea) family. It's used as a substitute for cocoa and chocolate because it doesn't have caffeine. It is high in insoluble and soluble fiber and is a rich source of antioxidants called polyphenols. A study in the *Journal of Nutrition* suggests that the insoluble fiber and antioxidants in carob can reduce food intake by decreasing levels of a hormone called ghrelin. Carob doesn't taste as bitter as cocoa, so less sugar is needed.

Shirataki noodles (pronounced shee-rah-*tah*-kee), also called kon-nyaku, sirataki, or yam noodles), are a type of Japanese noodle that has become extremely popular with dieters in North America. Derived from the root of the elephant yam or konjac plant, native to Asia, these white, gelatinous noodles are nearly all fiber, have only 20 calories per serving, and have no cholesterol, fat, or sugar, and only a few carbohydrates. The primary component is the soluble fiber glucomannan, which promotes weight loss because it soaks up water and physically expands in the stomach, helping you feel full. Glucomannan may also control appetite by increasing the level of hormones in the gut, such as cholecystokinin.

Shirataki noodles are almost flavorless and typically look like clear angel hair noodles, although there are now many shapes available. They usually come packed in liquid and should be refrigerated but not frozen. The noodles need to be rinsed well because they have a fishy odor even though they are not made with fish.

Some manufacturers add tofu to the noodles, so that they look and taste more like Italian pasta, but that adds some calories. Although cooking isn't necessary, boiling the noodles for a few minutes softens them (many people find them to have a rubbery consistency). After boiling, I find that rinsing them with cool water before adding them to sauces and other ingredients gives the best color and texture to dishes. Shirataki noodles can be found online and in the refrigerated section of some grocery and health food stores. Look in the tofu section in the produce aisle.

Another option is glucomannan, or konjac-mannan, powder. It is derived from konjac flour, like shirataki noodles. Studies have found that people who take glucomannan lose more weight than those who take a placebo. For example, in one eight-week double-blind study, people who were more than 20 percent over their ideal weight took 1 gram of glucomannan or a placebo 3 times a day, but were told not to change their eating or exercise habits. The people taking glucomannan had a significant average weight loss of 5.5 pounds and a reduction of total and LDL cholesterol and triglyceride levels, while those taking the placebo gained an average of 1.5 pounds.

If you are considering trying glucomannan, I suggest the powder and not the tablets. Because glucomannan absorbs water and expands, there have been several cases of throat obstruction with the tablets.

Get Enough Good Bacteria

The digestive tract of a healthy person has about 2 to 5 pounds of bacteria. Most are essential for our health, but some are potentially harmful. Maintaining a healthy balance of friendly versus unfriendly bacteria in the intestines is important to our weight and to our health. Too much unfriendly bacteria can stimulate cells in the liver called kupffer cells to release a chemical called tumor necrosis factor-alpha (TNF-alpha). TNF-alpha is involved in systemic inflammation, which puts an extra burden on the body and can lead to leptin and insulin resistance and weight gain.

One of the best ways to improve the balance of intestinal bacteria is with "probiotics," beneficial bacteria found in yogurt, sauerkraut, and a cultured milk beverage called kefir. Literally translated to mean "pro life," the use of probiotics dates back to the early twentieth century when Nobel Prize–winning researcher Elie Metchnikoff, director of the Pasteur Institute in Paris, noted that Bulgarian peasants who regularly consumed fermented foods containing beneficial bacteria had the greatest health and lived to an old age. Metchnikoff elaborated on his theory, known as the intoxication theory of aging, and advanced the belief that harmful intestinal bacteria released age-accelerating toxins and that eating probiotic foods could help to prevent that, which we now know to be true.

Beneficial bacteria also help with the detoxification of estrogenlike chemicals. Normally in the second step of detoxification, glucuronic acid is attached to the estrogen molecule so it can pass through bile into the colon. An enzyme in the colon called beta-glucuronidase, which is increased by a high-meat or high-fat diet, can split off the glucuronic acid molecule, allowing estrogen to sneak back and be reabsorbed. Probiotics and fiber keep this from happening by inhibiting the beta-glucuronidase enzyme.

Although you may be very familiar with yogurt, there is promising research about kefir, a milk drink that is cultured with beneficial yeast and bacteria. A Japanese study found that kefir reduces intestinal permeability and can inhibit yeast as well as other unwanted bacteria such as clostridia and enterobacteraciae from overgrowing in the colon.

Kefir is becoming quite popular, and it can be found in an increasing number of grocery stores in the yogurt section. It tastes rather tangy. I like to mix it with yogurt, another source of friendly bacteria, and have it with berries. You can also dilute it and have it as a healthier milk substitute.

How to Do It: Starting from step 2, have at least one serving (½ cup) of yogurt or kefir each day. Look for a product that says "active" or "live active cultures" on the label. Enjoy yogurt in a bowl topped with fresh berries and flaxseeds, or make a smoothie by putting ½ cup of yogurt in a blender with ½ cup of water, ¾ cup of berries, and 1 scoop of vanilla whey protein powder. For a super-fast smoothie, mix ¼ cup of unsweetened pomegranate or blueberry juice and a single-serving container of low-fat vanilla yogurt in a glass and stir until smooth.

Another option is strained yogurt. It has a thicker consistency than regular yogurt. A company called Fage makes a popular Greek strained yogurt called Total Yogurt that comes in a nonfat version that is thick and creamy, almost like cream cheese. You can also make your own by scooping plain, low-fat yogurt into a sieve lined with a double layer of cheesecloth and placing it over a bowl. Fold the ends of the cheesecloth over the sieve or use foil to cover it. Allow the yogurt to drain until it reaches the desired thickness. Scrape the yogurt from the cheesecloth and store it covered in the fridge. If you let it sit until it is very thick, you can add fresh herbs or garlic for a savory spread and use it instead of butter, cream cheese, or sour cream. You can also add lemon zest, vanilla extract, or cinnamon and serve it with sliced apples or other fruit.

If you are sensitive to dairy and can't eat yogurt or kefir, or if you have digestive problems or other health conditions and could benefit from a heftier dose of beneficial bacteria, try probiotic supplements, which come in vitamin bottles. Look for them in the refrigerated section at the health food store. Some of the better-known strains are lactobacillus and bifidobacteria. These supplements should be stored in your fridge. A typical dose is one to three capsules a day on an empty stomach. *Note:* Probiotics shouldn't be taken two weeks before or after surgery.

Sauerkraut is another probiotic food. There is a simple recipe for sauerkraut in the recipe section of this book that also contains anthocyanins from red cabbage.

Drink Enough Water

Making sure you drink enough water is one of the most basic and simple things you can do to cleanse your colon and detoxify your body. Our bodies need water. We are composed of over 70 percent water. Many of us are chronically dehydrated and walk around tired, weak, and hungry because of it. Not drinking enough water can also slow down metabolism.

Although ordinarily we get water from food and may not have to drink quite so much, we need to drink more water when we are trying to lose weight, which is why I suggest you strive for at least eight glasses a day. Drinking enough water can assist your efforts to slim down in the following ways:

- Diminishes hunger
- Improves metabolism
- Prevents constipation and improves digestive health
- Removes metabolic waste from the body, preventing body imbalances from developing
- Prevents the formation of cellulite
- Reduces stress (dehydration activates stress hormones) and stress-related cravings and abdominal weight gain

Try these ideas to gain the most benefit from the water you drink:

- Sip water slowly rather than gulping it. If you try to get your day's worth in one shot, it's likely to end up passing through you rather than being absorbed into your cells. You'll end up having to go to the bathroom every half hour.
- Avoid drinking water with meals. One glass is okay, but any more than that and it may be interfering with the digestion of your meal.
- Drink water at room temperature or warm. Water that's too hot or ice cold can impair digestion and hurt the fragile digestive lining.
- Flavor your water. Add a splash of lemon or lime juice.
- If you're used to drinking sodas and miss the sparkly fresh taste, try substituting carbonated spring water. Poland Spring's natural lemon-flavored spring water is quite good.
- You can count noncaffeinated herbal tea, vegetable juice, or soup toward your daily intake.
- Drink filtered water.

Water Filters

Typical tap water may contain runoff from industrial chemicals, heavy metals, solvents, excess copper from water pipes, chlorine, and PCBs.

Instead of drinking straight tap water, I suggest a solid carbon-block filter. With this filter, water is forced through a compressed carbon block. These water filters remove many chemicals, such as pesticides and organic chemicals, but their capabilities vary by brand, so it's important to check. One good-quality product is the Multi-Pure solid carbon-block filter. It removes PCBs and other chemicals, a claim that is certified by the National Sanitation Foundation International, a nonprofit testing lab.

Solid carbon-block filters are more effective at filtering water than are granular activated-carbon filters. Although the latter are the most popular household water filters (e.g., Brita) and remove any unpleasant tastes from water, less carbon comes in contact with water so they don't filter as well. Another popular but more expensive type of water filter is reverse osmosis. Many people find reverse osmosis systems too slow for regular household use, and they waste about five gallons of water for each gallon of filtered water.

Bottled Water

More than 40 percent of bottled waters come from municipal tap waters of cities like Wichita, Kansas; Queens, New York; and Jacksonville, Florida. Many bottlers add vitamins, minerals, flavorings, artificial sweeteners, and food color to enhance the flavor of the water, which makes it no better than diet soda. And despite its image, not all bottled water is cleaner than tap water. For example, in a study published in the journal *Archives of Family Medicine*, researchers compared fifty-seven samples of bottled water to tap water in Cleveland, Ohio, and found that thirty-nine of the bottled water samples were more pure than tap water, but fifteen of the bottled water samples had significantly more bacteria.

Bottled water also creates a lot of waste. The number of water bottles sold jumped from 3.3 billion in 1997 to 15 billion in 2002. The World Wildlife Fund estimates that 1.5 million tons of plastic are used each year around the world to make water bottles. According to the Container Recycling Institute, about 90 percent of plastic water bottles end up in landfills at a rate of thirty million a day. One plastic bottle can take up to a thousand years to break down. And finally, the manufacturing, transportation, and disposal of these bottles result in emissions that may ironically end up in our water.

. . .

How to Do It: Each day, drink at least eight glasses of filtered water. If you drink bottled water, a Colorado company called Biota was the first to make spring water bottled in a new type of biodegradable, compostable plastic called polylactic acid (PLA), made from corn, that will supposedly break down in just seventy-five to eighty days. Another Colorado company, New Wave Enviro Products, makes a PLA-based bottle that can be reused up to ninety times.

5

Restore Insulin and Leptin Sensitivity to Burn Fat

I burned sixty calories. That should take care of the peanut I had in 1962.

—ACTRESS RITA RUDNER

As you learned, insulin resistance changes the way that sugar and fat are metabolized in the liver, muscles, and fat cells. Insulin resistance encourages the formation of new fat in our waist, hips, and thighs, and also the hidden fat in the liver. It is difficult to burn the fat until cells become sensitive to insulin again.

The other big culprit, leptin resistance, disrupts our body's ability to regulate appetite and metabolism. As you're about to learn, the wrong foods can worsen the problem, and the right foods, which you'll find on the Inside Out Diet, can correct the problem, ensuring that these vital hormone messages get properly received through your system.

Include Healthy Oils

Bile can also get too thick if it's not emptied completely or often enough from the gallbladder. This often happens during weight loss, especially if your diet is too low in healthy fats, you skip meals, or go without eating for long periods. Eating healthy fats, in moderation, can prevent this because they promote the release of bile from the gallbladder. The best oils to use regularly in food are those rich in monounsaturated fats, because they can also lower the risk of heart disease and won't alter the balance of omega fatty acids.

Here are some favorite oils that are high in monounsaturated fats:

- *Olive oil* contains compounds called phenols that are anti-inflammatory and antioxidant. A study in the *Journal of the American College of Cardiology* found that extra-virgin olive oil has the highest phenol content. Olive oil phenols increase levels of a molecule called nitric oxide, which keeps blood vessels dilated and decreases free-radical damage, making it a liver healer. And it adds a delicious flavor to food!

- *Avocado oil* is extracted from the flesh of avocados, not the seed. It has a higher smoking point, even compared to that of olive oil and most nut oils, making it the top choice for sautés or stir-fries. The oil doesn't have much flavor, so it is quite versatile. Of course, an avocado on its own is delicious. Avocados also contain potassium (even more than bananas) and vitamin E and are cholesterol-free and low in saturated fats. They taste great with tomatoes, black olives, onions, fresh parsley, and cilantro. Try spreading some ripe avocado on toast; the creamy, buttery texture and flavor make it a great alternative to butter.

- *Macadamia nut oil* has a rich, nutty flavor that complements many dishes. It also has a higher smoking point, which makes it an ideal cooking oil. If you can't find it in the grocery store, look for it in specialty or health food stores.

- *Hazelnut oil* is a luscious, deeply flavored oil. Try drizzling it over salads, or pairing it with artichokes or wild rice. Blend it with a lighter-tasting oil, such as avocado or olive oil, to bring out the flavor.

- *Almond oil*, rich in vitamin E, has a clean flavor and can be used in cooking or in salad dressings, pesto, and other dishes. A study published in the *Journal of Nutrition* found that people who replaced half the fat in their diets with almonds or almond oil reduced total and LDL cholesterol by 4 percent and 6 percent respectively. Their triglycerides fell by 14 percent.

How to Do It: Replace old or unhealthy oils in your pantry with these healthy oils for use in cooking, seasoning, and salad dressings. Oil is rancid if it smells stale or has been sitting in your pantry for more than a year. Experiment with oils you have never tried before. Some really add depth and flavor. If you've avoided cooking with certain oils because they seem high in fat, not to worry. All oils have the same number of calories— 120 per tablespoon of oil (it's a very common misconception, though, that some oils are higher in calories than others). Some nuts, on the other hand, have a greater proportion of oil than other nuts, which is why the number of calories differs in nuts.

Avoid overheating oils. You should never heat oil to the point that it starts to smoke. An oil's smoking point is the temperature at which it burns. For example, the smoking point of extra-virgin olive oil is 320 degrees, whereas the smoking point of virgin olive oil is 420 degrees, which is why virgin olive oil is preferable for cooking. Heating an oil to its smoking point or beyond can generate harmful compounds.

When shopping for oils, look for those that have been minimally processed. When checking the label, look for the words "expeller-pressed" or "cold-pressed." After opening a new bottle of oil, squeeze one capsule of vitamin E oil into the bottle to keep it from going stale. Store oil in the refrigerator and let it sit for ten minutes at room temperature before using it. Pour olive oil (you can also use grapeseed or avocado oil) into a spray bottle so you can reduce the amount used during cooking. Many recipes in this book use olive oil spray.

Avoid vegetable oils such as corn, safflower, sunflower, and cottonseed. Although these are the most prevalent oils, they actually alter our omega fatty-acid balance so we end up with too much omega-6 fatty acids and a relative deficiency of omega-3 fatty acids. Check labels, because these oils are found in most processed foods, including cookies, breads, muffins, cakes, chips, and other commercial snack foods.

Stay away from foods that have the words "trans fat" on the label. If you must eat them, choose brands that contain as little as possible, because no amount is good for you. Trans fats were invented in the 1940s, when food manufacturers figured out that by heating polyunsaturated vegetable oil and steeping it with hydrogen, they could make the oil solid and spreadable at room temperature and extend the shelf life of processed foods. Trans fats are used in many baked goods or snack foods that sit on supermarket shelves, including breads, crackers, cookies, muffins, and chips. They are now linked with an increased incidence of heart disease, Alzheimer's disease, diabetes, and certain cancers. Harvard University's

Nurses Health Study found that women who ate the most trans fats, about 3 percent of their food intake, were 50 percent more likely to develop heart disease. What's surprising is that 3 percent amounts to about 7 grams of trans fats, and many of us get far more than that every day.

Get Plenty of Omegas

Omega fatty acids are also called essential fats, because our bodies can't make them by themselves but must obtain them through diet or else we become deficient. Omega fatty-acid deficiency is very common today, resulting in systemic, low-grade inflammation that can lead to insulin and leptin resistance and weight gain. Omega fatty-acid deficiency has also been linked with heart disease, depression, rheumatoid arthritis, skin disorders, and inflammatory bowel disease. Signs of deficiency include dry or rough skin, brittle or soft nails, dry hair, and dandruff.

There are two main types of omega fatty acids—omega-3 and omega-6. We require both. The biologically active forms of omega-3 are EPA (eicosapentaenoic acid) and DHA (docosahexaenoic acid). Our main animal source is cold-water fish, which you already learned isn't a great choice because it comes loaded with unwanted chemicals. Plant sources such as flaxseed oil, walnuts, green leafy vegetables, and soybeans are in a form that must be converted in our bodies to the active forms, but diets high in saturated fats, trans fats, and sugar can block the formation of active omega-3s from these precursors. High insulin levels, stress, aging, hypothyroidism, vitamin deficiency, and illness can also interfere. As a result, we only consume an estimated 130 mg of these active omega-3s a day, at least 520 mg less than the minimum 650 mg recommended by an international panel of essential fatty-acid experts.

By far, the main sources of omega-6s in our food supply are from vegetable oils such as corn oil, safflower oil, and sunflower oil. A small amount gets converted into healthy omega-6s called GLA (gamma linolenic acid). Like the omega-3s, poor diet and illness lessen this conversion.

What's key here is the balance. The earliest human diet had an ideal omega-3 to omega-6 ratio of 1 to 1. What's considered an optimal ratio to strive for today is 1 to 5 or less. In the past century, there has been a huge increase in omega-6 in our diets, largely because omega-6 vegetable oils, which include corn oil, safflower oil, and sunflower oil, are relatively cheap to produce. They're found in most processed foods, including cookies, breads, muffins, cakes, chips, and other commercial snack foods. As a result, we've moved far from the ideal, and what's typical nowadays is an omega-3 to omega-6 ratio of 1 to 20.

When the omega-6 level gets too high, as it is for most of us, two unfortunate things happen:

1. More proinflammatory arachidonic acid is made. Arachidonic acids are precursors to a group of prostaglandins that promotes inflammation and adversely affects the heart.
2. Less of the omega-3 precursors get converted to active omega-3, because they compete for the same enzyme also needed for the vegetable oil-to-arachidonic acid conversion.

More and more studies are showing that a higher intake of omega-6 with a low intake of omega-3 is a major cause of inflammation and is the reason why the incidence of inflammatory diseases, including heart disease, is skyrocketing.

Why Omega-3 Fats Are Essential during Weight Loss

Some of the specific benefits of omega-3 fats during weight loss include the following:

• *Raise our metabolic rate and helps us burn fat.* Animals fed an omega-3-rich diet had a reduction in the size and number of fat cells. A study published in *Physiology Research* randomly assigned women classified as having severe obesity to a placebo diet or a diet supplemented with omega-3 fats. Researchers analyzed both groups and found that the omega-3-supplemented diet resulted in a significantly greater reduction in weight, body mass index, and hip circumference compared to the other group. Another study looked at what would happen when omega-3 fats were deficient, which is the case for many of us. An omega-3-deficient diet resulted in increased body fat and impaired glucose tolerance.

• *Keep cell membranes healthy and fluid so cells can communicate with one another.* Omega-3s are also a crucial part of cell membranes. If we don't have enough omega-3s, our cell membranes become rigid and cannot properly receive messages sent by our hormones and the appetite-influencing neurotransmitters serotonin and dopamine.

- *Prevent gallstone formation during weight loss.* Gallstones are often formed when people try to lose weight. A study published in the *Journal of Nutrition* looked at the effect of omega-3s on cholesterol saturation of bile in people who were trying to lose weight. After six weeks, the researchers found that cholesterol saturation had increased significantly in the placebo group and the group taking medication to prevent gallstones but not in the omega-3 group.

- *Restore leptin sensitivity.* Omega fatty acids are one of the key ways we can restore leptin sensitivity. By reducing inflammation, they improve cell membrane function, allowing cells to hear leptin's messages and keep off those unwanted pounds.

- *Are vital for detoxification.* Not having enough omega-3s is linked to excess inflammation, because it alters the balance of unwanted prostaglandins. The inflammation and free radicals disrupt cell membranes, allowing toxins to leak in, damaging DNA, enzymes, protein synthesis, and mitochondrial function. This is heightened during weight loss due to the increased exposure to toxins.

- *Lower triglycerides and suppresses the formation of liver fat.* In a review of human studies, omega-3 fats were found to inhibit the synthesis of triglycerides in people with high triglycerides. A Penn State study concurred, reporting that dietary omega-3 fats decreased the risk of heart disease by lowering inflammatory markers. The omega-3 fats also reduced total cholesterol, LDL cholesterol, and triglycerides and increased good HDL cholesterol. Omega-3 fatty acids also appear to suppress the accumulation of fat in the liver.

- *Reduce the risk of heart disease.* Omega-3 fats have been widely studied for their effects on the heart. They've been found to lower inflammation in arteries, stabilize plaque, and decrease the risk of heart attack, stroke, and sudden death from heart arrhythmias. In fact, in 2002, the American Heart Association recommended that people with heart disease increase their intake of omega-3s to 1 gram of combined EPA and DHA a day.

How to Do It: Consider taking an omega fatty-acid supplement one to three times a day. The most beneficial type of omega fatty-acid supplement for weight loss and overall health is one that contains all three of the active omega fatty acids—EPA, DHA, and GLA—from a mixture of fish oil plus evening primrose, black currant, or borage seed oils. The ratio is important, and the ideal ratio of omega-3 (EPA and DHA) to omega-6 (GLA) is 5:1. For example, one capsule would contain 150 mg EPA, 100 mg DHA, and 50 mg GLA.

One brand you may wish to look into is Nordic Naturals, which uses a technique called molecular distillation to filter out toxins from the fish oil. The company makes a product called ProEFA, which contains the 5-to-1 ratio. Whatever brand you choose, take it just before meals. Fish oil has a mild blood-thinning effect, so people taking blood-thinning medication or who are at risk of bleeding complications should check with their doctor before taking omega fatty acids. If you are allergic to fish, substitute with 1 tablespoon of flaxseed oil per day.

Eat Foods with a Lower Glycemic Load

Though I've made little distinction between the types of carbohydrates so far, one is very important: certain carbohydrates are better than others at setting off the insulin surge. By eating the right carbohydrates, we can reduce our need for insulin.

We used to think of carbs as being just simple or complex based on their chemical structure. Simple carbohydrates were sugars, whereas complex carbohydrates were long chains of linked sugars that had to be broken down. But this turned out to be an overly simplistic way of classifying carbs, because it didn't predict their impact on blood sugar and insulin. For example, white rice (complex) and sugar (simple) cause a similar surge in these markers.

The Glycemic Index

In 1981, David Jenkins, M.D., and his colleagues at the University of Toronto published a study introducing a more precise system of classifying carbs called the glycemic index (GI). You may have heard of it before. It's been used in many popular diets to distinguish "good" and "bad" carbohydrates. The so-called "good" carbohydrates release their sugar slowly, supplying energy at a steady level throughout the day. The "bad" high-GI carbs are digested quickly, which means that your energy soon plunges, causing cravings and tiredness.

What Dr. Jenkins and his colleagues did was rank carbs numerically according to how quickly they were absorbed into the bloodstream.

Glucose is used as a benchmark and given a score of 100. Some foods break down quickly, causing a dramatic rise; these foods have a higher score, or GI. Lower numbers mean the food is converted into sugar more slowly.

Looking through this brief list, you'll notice that potatoes rank at 85, because the starch converts to blood sugar easily. Plain bagels also score relatively high, as do cookies, chips, breakfast cereals, soft drinks, and other refined carbohydrates, whereas higher-fiber foods such as green beans and other vegetables, fruits, and beans take longer to digest and have a slower release of sugar into the blood.

Food	GI Score	Food	GI Score
White bread	70	Grapefruit	25
Crisp rice cereal	87	Watermelon	72
Bagel	72	Tomato	<20
Corn flakes	92	Carrots	49
White rice	72	Potato, baked	85
Mars bar	68	Potato chips	57
Breton wheat crackers	67	Green beans	<20

Because the GI allows you to determine how much a certain food will impact your blood sugar, I'm sure you can appreciate how valuable a tool this can be compared to the simple-versus-complex classification. Study after study confirms it. For example, the Harvard Nurses Health Study of seventy-five thousand women found that those who consumed high glycemic-index diets had double the incidence of heart disease and 40 percent more diabetes than those eating diets based on lower glycemic-index foods. Higher glycemic-index foods eaten regularly also have been associated with increased risk of stroke.

As effective as it is, there's a problem that makes the glycemic index not so practical for us to use at home: it doesn't take into account the portion sizes we usually eat. For example, white bread has a GI of 70 and watermelon has a similar rating of 72. Going by the GI alone, they would be considered equivalent. However, 50 grams (the benchmark amount) of carbs from white bread is three slices, but to get 50 grams of carbs from watermelon, we'd need to eat an entire melon in one sitting!

Many popular diets overly relied on the GI without understanding this basic fact that some foods, like white bread, potatoes, and cakes, just naturally contain a larger amount of carbohydrate, while others, such as watermelon, apples, and carrots, contain relatively little. As a result, those diets were needlessly limited and you don't see watermelon on their list of healthy foods.

Glycemic Load versus Glycemic Index

It's also important to know about another system for classifying carbs called the glycemic load (GL), proposed by researchers at Harvard in 1997. It still uses the glycemic index, but the score gets multiplied by the number of carbs we're likely to eat in a normal serving.

The following list shows how glycemic load is more practical than the glycemic index in that it reveals how some carbs we thought of as "bad" are actually okay. Going back to our previous example, a more normal-size serving of one cup of watermelon would rate low on the GL at 8. By considering both the grams of carbohydrate in a typical serving and how quickly they're converted to blood sugar, this dual approach is less restrictive and can help people control their carb intake over the course of the day.

While it's important to generally eat foods that have a lower GL, keep in mind that the important thing to look at is the overall profile of the meal.

Food	GI	Grams of Carbs	GL
Apple	38	15	6
Grapes	46	18	8
Orange	48	11	5
Pumpkin	75	15	11
Peach	42	11	5
Sweet potato	61	27	16
Almonds	0	0	0
Ice cream	38	14	5
Bran flakes	74	18	13
White rice	72	36	26
Kidney beans	28	25	7
Carrots	49	5	2
Carrot juice	43	21	9
Watermelon	72	11	8
Multigrain bread	49	24	10
Pasta, whole wheat	42	38	16
Potato chips	57	18	10

Food	GI	Grams of Carbs	GL
Mashed potato	104	34	18
Bagel	72	56	40
White bread	70	24	17

Low GI = 55 or less; moderate GI = 56 to 59; high GI = 70 or more.
Low GL = 10 or less; moderate GL = 11 to 19; high GL = 20 or more.

What Are Some Lower-Glycemic Starchy Foods?

I've handpicked some lower-glycemic foods that are especially good for your liver. These foods are detoxifying and packed with nutrients, which will help satisfy hunger and promote weight loss:

- *Barley.* Barley is a great food for detoxifying and losing weight because, like oats, it's an excellent source of soluble fiber, which further helps to lower cholesterol, stabilize blood sugar, and reduce hunger between meals. Pearled barley, the most popular kind, has a pleasant, chewy texture that makes it a good substitute for rice. To save time, look for quick-cooking pearled barley, which has been precooked by steaming. Barley grits make a delicious hot breakfast cereal.

- *Brown rice.* Brown rice retains the bran layer, which is packed with vitamins and minerals, such as niacin, vitamin B6, and magnesium. It has four times the amount of insoluble fiber as white rice. Quick-cooking brown rice is now available, which has been precooked so that it can be reheated in minutes. Studies by the Fukuoka Institute of Health and Environmental Sciences in Japan have found that brown rice is particularly good at enhancing the elimination of PCBs and other chemicals from the body.

- *Buckwheat.* Buckwheat contains relatively high levels of d-chiro-inositol, a compound that has been found to lower blood glucose in animals and is showing promise as a treatment for diabetes. Toasted buckwheat groats, also known as kasha, have an intense, hearty taste, and it can be eaten alone or mixed with rice for a milder flavor. You can also find unroasted buckwheat groats, which are pale and bland, which makes them a good rice alternative. Despite its name, buckwheat isn't related to wheat and isn't a true grain but a fruit. It has a relatively short cooking time of approximately fifteen minutes. Some cookbooks suggest beating an egg white into the kernels before adding the water to make the buckwheat light and fluffy.

- *Cauliflower.* I like cauliflower because it's one of the few cruciferous vegetables that can be used as a substitute for starchy foods. Cauliflower can be chopped finely in the food processor to simulate the texture of rice or it can be mashed like potatoes.

- *Peas.* Peas contain soluble fiber. Try heating frozen peas in the microwave and mixing them with brown rice and ground flaxseeds.

- *Quinoa.* Quinoa, pronounced *keen-wa*, has a light, delicate taste and, unlike most whole grains, it cooks quickly. It is the seed of a plant that originated in the Andes in South America. Quinoa contains 50 percent more protein than most other grains. It is also a complete protein, providing all eight essential amino acids. In fact, the World Health Organization rated the quality of quinoa's protein as equivalent to milk. Although the seeds are small, they expand with cooking until they are fluffy. When it's cooked, a tiny, opaque spiral appears on the grain, which curls to the center and is pleasantly crunchy. Quinoa should be rinsed well before cooking to remove any residues of the protective bitter coating.

- *Red lentils.* Dried red lentils take only twenty minutes to cook. They cook faster than any other bean or legume and do not require presoaking. Add cooked lentils to brown rice, quinoa, buckwheat, or other grains.

- *Spaghetti squash.* Large, yellow spaghetti squash looks like any other squash when you slice open a raw one. But once it's cooked, the flesh pulls away in thin strands resembling spaghetti. It can be used as a nonstarchy spaghetti substitute. Spaghetti squash is low in calories and an excellent source of potassium, magnesium, and vitamin C. To cook spaghetti squash, pierce it with a fork and bake it whole until tender. Allow it to cool slightly and cut it in half. Discard the seeds and pulp, and scrape the flesh into a bowl.

Best Beans

The key to eating beans without causing a scene is to introduce them slowly into your diet. You may also wish to use Beano or another enzyme supplement to help digest them.

Lentils and split peas are less gas-producing than larger beans and legumes and don't need to be presoaked. Canned beans are a time-saving option, but be sure to rinse them thoroughly to remove the excess salt.

- *Sweet potato.* Sweet potatoes are a rich source of both beta-carotene and vitamin C. What's really unique about sweet potatoes is that preliminary studies have found a compound in sweet potatoes that helps to stabilize blood sugar and insulin. It also slows the absorption of sugar because it contains soluble fiber.

- *Turnips.* Like cauliflower, turnips are a cruciferous vegetable that can be mashed and used instead of potatoes. They also have about a third of the calories of potatoes.

- *Wild rice.* Wild rice has a dark color, a rich, nutty flavor, and a chewy texture. This long, black grass is native to North America. It contains more protein than brown or white rice. You can mix it with brown rice or into salads. It should be rinsed well before cooking. Wild rice takes about fifty minutes to cook. When done, it becomes puffy and splits open.

How to Do It: Try to eat these weight-loss-friendly, lower-glycemic grains and starchy foods instead of white rice, crackers, bread, pasta, muffins, fries, and chips, which trigger hunger and weight gain. You don't have to try these new foods all at once. Gradually add them to your diet, allowing yourself time to experiment and grow to appreciate the new flavors.

Any grain can be lightly toasted in the pot before boiling. It adds a delicious roasted flavor to the grain. For example, gently toast rice in the same pot you're going to boil it in. After it's toasted, just add the water and boil as usual. Use this as a transition if you are starting to eat whole grains, because toasting slightly raises the glycemic load of the grain and can affect the quality of the oil in the grain.

If you aren't quite ready to make the transition from white to brown rice, try adding some ground flaxseeds to white rice. The added fiber lowers the glycemic load of the meal.

Add a Dash of Cinnamon

This popular spice appears to have an insulinlike effect and increases a cell's ability to use glucose. It can significantly help people normalize their blood sugar levels. Just one-quarter to one-half teaspoon can result in a 20 percent drop in blood sugar. A study found that having one-half teaspoon a day for nearly six weeks reduced blood levels of glucose and triglycerides, and reduced LDL cholesterol by almost 20 percent.

Cinnamon also tastes sweet, so you can use it to decrease your intake of sugar. The active compounds aren't destroyed by heat. *Note*: Cinnamon contains coumarin, which in larger amounts can have a blood-thinning effect. Consult your doctor first if you are taking the drug warfarin or are at risk of bleeding complications for any reason.

How to Do It: Drink Cleansing Lemon Tea (see page 223), which has cinnamon in it. Try adding a dash of cinnamon instead of sugar to foods, such as desserts, to take advantage of cinnamon's naturally sweet flavor.

Consider Using Natural Sweeteners

You'll notice that you quickly lose your cravings on the Inside Out Diet. But when you do wish to add sweetness to food, consider trying these natural sweeteners.

- *Erythritol.* Erythritol is a sugar alcohol that has about 70 percent of the sweetness of table sugar but has almost zero calories and carbohydrates. It doesn't affect blood sugar and doesn't cause bloating and digestive upset like other sugar alcohols (e.g., sorbitol), because most of it (between 60 and 90 percent) is absorbed in the small intestine and later excreted in urine. It has a cool, mildly sweet taste. Erythritol is found naturally in small amounts in fruit, mushrooms, and fermented drinks such as wine. Powdered erythritol is available. Most companies manufacture it from the fermentation of cornstarch. Erythritol is approved for use in the United States.

- *Luo han guo.* A small light green fruit grown in southern China, luo han guo fruit (*Momordica grosvenorii, Siraitia grosvenorii*) is often called a longevity fruit in Asia. It is used there as a natural sweetener due to its lack of calories, and like stevia, luo han guo is three hundred times sweeter than sugar. The sweet taste is due to compounds called triterpene glycosides, which have been found to suppress the rise in blood glucose after meals and inhibit the oxidation of LDL cholesterol.

- *Rapadura and sucanat.* Made from sugar cane juice (same as white sugar), rapadura and sucanat are much more flavorful and satisfying (meaning you'll consume less) than white sugar because they haven't been refined. For instance, rapadura is sugar cane that has been boiled to remove the water. It's even less processed than evaporated cane juice, another sweetener. Both have a toffee, molasseslike flavor and contain vitamins and minerals. These sweeteners should be used sparingly anywhere sugar is used. Keep in mind that they'll affect the color and flavor of certain foods.

- *Stevia.* Stevia is a plant native to Paraguay that contains a naturally sweet substance called stevioside. Commercial stevia extracts were first developed in Japan in the 1970s. The powdered extract looks like white sugar, contains zero calories, and is three hundred times sweeter than sugar. Although Japanese studies suggest it is a safe sugar substitute, there haven't been many studies conducted in the United States so it is not approved by the FDA as a sugar substitute. Two studies in rats found that stevia lowered male sperm counts, but no study has yet confirmed if this finding also holds true for humans. Researchers in Denmark found that stevioside reduced postmeal blood glucose levels in type 2 diabetic patients, suggesting that stevia, unlike other sweeteners, may have a beneficial effect on glucose metabolism.

  Stevia can be found in health food stores, some grocery stores, and online. It comes in powder or liquid form, and either can be added to food and beverages. Stevia products naturally taste slightly bitter, but the bitterness is mostly removed during processing.

- *Yacon syrup.* A dark brown syrup that has a molasseslike taste, yacon syrup is made from a tuber that grows in the Andes in South America. Yacon root is naturally sweet-tasting and low calorie because it contains carbohydrates called oligofructans. The human body lacks the enzymes to metabolize oligofructans, which means that although they taste sweet, they pass through the digestive tract without raising blood glucose or calories. The oligofructans are prebiotics, which mean they support the growth of beneficial bacteria such as lactobacillus and bifidobacteria in the colon. Although yacon syrup is a promising sweetener, preliminary studies suggest that after harvesting the yacon root, some of the oligofructans are converted into the sugars fructose, glucose, and sucrose, especially if the root is subjected to high heat and sunlight. Using raw yacon syrup (and not cooking with it) may reduce the conversion.

Avoid Fructose Sweeteners

Fructose is a simple sugar found naturally in honey, fruit, and some root vegetables such as beets and sweet potatoes. Sweeteners that contain high amounts of fructose, such as honey, agave nectar, fruit concentrates, and high-fructose corn syrup may be just as bad as, if not worse than, regular white sugar (sucrose).

Fructose was promoted as a healthy sweetener because it has a minimal effect on blood sugar and insulin levels; however, it also doesn't influence the levels of leptin or ghrelin, hormones involved in appetite regulation, so it may increase food intake. Fructose is also converted into triglycerides more readily than sucrose and is stored as fat. Fructose is metabolized by the liver, and eating an amount that exceeds the liver's capacity to oxidize it can lead to fatty liver.

Although the fructose in fruit and small amounts of juice are acceptable and provide antioxidants and soluble fiber, fructose-based sweeteners are more concentrated and should be avoided.

6

Check for Food Intolerances

Tell me what you eat, and I'll tell you what you are.
—FRENCH LAWYER AND GASTRONOMIST ANTHELME BRILLAT-SAVARIN

My client Leslie, an elementary school teacher, was on the verge of tears. She had come to me because she was experiencing cravings and bloating and had steadily gained eleven pounds in the past year and a half.

"It's so embarrassing. When I'm talking with my students, I hear my stomach starting to rumble. I'm so worried I'm going to pass gas in front of the class. Some days, I feel like a balloon ready to pop!"

When I looked over Leslie's diet diary, I immediately recognized a pattern I see quite often. Leslie inhaled her lunch during the few minutes she had in between morning classes and coaching the girls' tennis team at lunch. Her meals usually contained cheese ("I can't live without it!"), ham, and bread, all washed down by a glass of skim milk. She often ate a diet snack on the way home.

I explained to Leslie that stress, hurried eating, and the foods she was relying on day after day were disrupting the balance of bacteria in her gut, causing inflammation of her intestinal wall and making her crave and react to foods she had no trouble with before. I told her that this easily corrected imbalance can result in intense cravings and make her gain weight.

Although Leslie was experiencing digestive problems, more than 50 percent of people with food reactions don't have any digestive symptoms whatsoever. You could be one of them. The only symptoms may be cravings and difficulty losing weight.

Leslie agreed to try the diet, even though she was hesitant about having to give up her beloved cheese. Three weeks after starting it, she stopped by my office for an appointment. She said, "This is the first time in two years I haven't been bloated! My stomach is flat again!" Her incessant cravings had diminished, and water that was locked away in her tissues was markedly reduced. Unencumbered by the reactive foods that were causing inflammation in her intestines, her metabolism could start to repair itself.

Food Intolerances Can Overload the Liver

Many people think of their immune system as something that fights off respiratory infections, but by far the largest and most active part of our immune system is our digestive tract, which is over thirty feet long. Over 80 percent of our antibody-producing cells are made there, and 50 percent of our lymph tissue is in the intestines. Bacteria, viruses, chemicals, toxins, waste, and undigested foods make their way into our digestive tract every day and can't be allowed to get absorbed in our bloodstream. If they are, they have to go to the liver to be detoxified. The digestive barrier, therefore, has many guards, including stomach acid, digestive enzymes, beneficial bacteria, and very selective, narrow pores.

Anything that causes irritation or damage can over time weaken the thin gut barrier, and the result is that those unwanted substances can sneak through the widened pores and into the bloodstream. An extra burden is placed on the liver to process this material. The body reacts to these unwanted substances, triggering an inflammatory response. If the unwanted substance is undigested food, it is called a food reaction.

You probably know someone who has a severe allergy to nuts, shellfish, or another food. Unlike out-and-out food allergies that trigger immediate, life-threatening reactions such as anaphylactic shock, difficulty breathing, and throat swelling, these hidden, delayed food reactions are more likely to result in weight gain, cravings, low energy, bloating, indigestion, and other more subtle symptoms. They're usually not evident unless they're specifically unmasked through testing.

Food intolerances place a great demand on the liver and can result in cravings and a number of problems related to weight:

- Inflammation causes a vicious cycle, interfering with the ability of cells to respond to leptin and preventing glucose from entering cells. We end up overeating and craving sugary foods, which only worsens the inflammation. More toxins can sneak through the now-compromised intestinal barrier, leading to further weight gain.
- The ever-present barrage of bacteria, viruses, and chemicals that a weakened intestinal barrier has to block puts a great stress on the body. Cortisol rises, resulting in increased blood sugar and a corresponding rise in insulin. Because this burden is continuous and such a large part of our body is being threatened, blood sugar and insulin remain elevated. As a result, we store more fat. The elevated cortisol also makes us hungry.
- Removal of the trigger foods usually results in a rapid loss of five or more pounds of water that was locked away in body tissues. It can dramatically reduce puffiness, swelling, and bloating. More important, following the initial release from our waterlogged tissues, removal of the offending foods allows the person to burn fat.

A Whole Set of Health Issues

Most people don't realize that delayed food reactions have been implicated in a wide range of seemingly unrelated symptoms and conditions, from indigestion to arthritis, diabetes, depression, and chronic fatigue syndrome. Because digestive symptoms only occur in 50 percent of people, food intolerances are often not considered.

Even when digestive symptoms are present, many people don't appreciate the significant role food reactions can play in health.

Digestive

Bloating and gas	Ulcerative colitis
Diarrhea	Irritable bowel syndrome
Abdominal pain and cramps	Celiac disease
Constipation	Candida

Endocrine

| Thyroid disease | Insulin resistance | Diabetes |

Skin

Acne	Rash
Canker sores	Hives, itching
Eczema	

Neurological

Headache	Migraines
Fatigue	Depression
Insomnia	Anxiety

Muscle and Joint

| Joint pain | Bursitis |
| Chronic muscle pain | |

Autoimmune

| Rheumatoid arthritis | Lupus |
| Multiple sclerosis | |

Respiratory

| Chronic cough | Postnasal drip |
| Chronic bronchitis | Chronic sinus congestion |

Zoltan Rona, M.D., notes that mineral deficiencies often occur because carrier proteins in the intestinal wall that are needed to properly absorb minerals are damaged by inflammation, resulting in magnesium, zinc, copper, calcium, and other mineral deficiencies. This can lead to a worsening of cravings and further weight gain because many hormones involved in controlling weight rely on these minerals.

What Are Your Problem Foods?

It has been estimated that as many as 60 percent of all North Americans suffer from hidden food intolerances. The foods we tend to crave are very often the foods we're sensitive to. For example, the person who can't live without bread or pasta can be sensitive to wheat, or the person who loves cheese may have a dairy sensitivity. There is intriguing research showing

Attention, Chocoholics

Did you know that a hidden magnesium deficiency may be making you crave chocolate? A mere ounce of baker's chocolate contains 87 mg of this necessary mineral.

Magnesium is an extremely important mineral, the second most predominant mineral after potassium in our cells. Some of magnesium's main functions are to activate enzymes, such as those involved in detoxification. Decreased magnesium levels have been linked to nonalcoholic steatohepatitis (NASH).

The average intake of magnesium is less than 266 mg per day, far below what is recommended. Symptoms of magnesium deficiency include muscle cramping, headaches, constipation, insomnia, PMS, menstrual cramps, high blood pressure, and a tendency to get stressed. There is also a relationship between decreased magnesium levels in blood and insulin resistance.

that particles of problem foods such as milk and wheat pass through the intestinal lining, stimulating opiate receptor sites and boosting serotonin levels, which make us feel better for a short time after we eat these foods. As the good feeling wears off, we're left feeling worse until we eat the food again. That's why we have powerful cravings for the foods we're sensitive to.

Most people have no idea this is going on until they eliminate the food from their diet and later test it. It's quite common to experience signs of withdrawal in the first week, such as cravings, anxiety, and a mild headache. The majority of food reactions is caused by just two trigger foods: milk and milk products and wheat.

Casein, the protein in milk, has been shown to have morphinelike activity in the body, which is why it is also called casomorphin. This addictive property serves a biological purpose in those it's intended for— newborn mammals. A newborn's only form of sustenance is mother's milk, so it must quickly develop a strong liking for it and continue to want it until it is old enough to find its own food. In fact, all milk, even human breast milk, has casomorphins.

People also have trouble digesting the lactose sugar in milk. Babies can, but as they get older, most lose the enzyme lactase, which is needed to break down the lactose, because there is no longer any need for them to rely on breast milk. In fact, three-quarters of adults in the world are lactose intolerant. In the United States, 75 percent of African Americans, 50 percent of Hispanic Americans, and 90 percent of Asian Americans have some difficulty digesting lactose. Although these figures are informative, in my practice I've found milk to be the most common food reaction regardless of cultural heritage. It can affect anyone.

Obvious signs are bloating, cramps, gas, diarrhea, and nausea. But more frequently, there aren't any obvious symptoms, just subtle signs of a sensitivity, like nasal or sinus congestion, postnasal drip, constipation, heartburn, and cravings that can only be unmasked with testing.

How to Do It: You need to figure out what foods may be causing problems for you. In the first week of the Inside Out Diet, you'll eliminate certain foods. During the second week, you'll reintroduce them into your diet and note in a journal how your body responds. It's a quick and easy check to help you gauge whether foods that you normally eat may be giving you cravings or making you feel bloated, tired, sluggish, or worse. This test is not used for any foods that you already know you are allergic to or foods that cause immediate reactions. It's only to look for more subtle, delayed reactions that affect us. It's based on elimination and challenge, a method used for decades as a way to help people find out whether certain foods are contributing to their health problems. It's widely considered to be the gold standard, confirmed by a report in the journal *American Family Physician*: "Most patients can be safely evaluated by a food elimination diet followed by a specific food challenge at home or in the office setting. At present, an appropriately performed challenge test is the definitive procedure for verifying a cause-and-effect relationship between exposure to a particular food and the appearance of certain symptoms or signs."

Caution: You should not try this test with any known food allergies. Do not eat any food you already know causes an allergy or is believed to be a possible cause of health problems. The purpose of this challenge is to uncover sensitivities to foods you eat frequently but that are not presently recognized as a possible cause of health problems. If any food has caused symptoms in the past, never test it without your doctor's advice. Do not try this test if you have asthma or celiac disease, if you use an EpiPen, are pregnant or nursing, have weakened immunity, or have symptoms that could harm you if they are temporarily aggravated, as your condition may temporarily worsen after a challenge. If you have chronic health problems, always start with a visit to your doctor.

You'll temporarily avoid the most common problematic foods in step 1, including dairy and wheat. After one week, you'll start adding them back (you can also choose to wait until the beginning of the third or fourth week before you add back foods if your symptoms haven't settled down). Each day, you'll add just one new test food as your midmorning snack, noting in a journal any reaction to it, such as unusual cravings, bloating, or other symptoms for the rest of the day and the following morning (see the sample journal on page 94). If you don't notice anything in those twenty-four hours, you can now eat that food as part of your step 2 plan, but wait until after the entire testing period before you eat it again. The exception is organic yogurt or kefir—because of its many health benefits, you can begin eating either food after the test day if you don't react to it.

If you experience symptoms after eating a food, don't add it back, however. If you wish, try halving the portion to see if you can tolerate a smaller amount. If it still causes symptoms, you should avoid that food altogether for now.

Which Foods? Here are the foods to try and suggested test amounts.

- Day 1: Organic yogurt or kefir, ½ cup
- Day 2: Cheese (any type of low-fat cheese), 1 ounce
- Day 3: Barley, ½ cup cooked
- Day 4: Whole wheat spaghetti, ½ cup
- Day 5: Rye bread, 1 slice
- Day 6: Skim milk, 1 cup
- Day 7: Whole grain bread, 1 slice

What to Look For: Your response will be entirely individual. Just pay attention to your body and the messages it's sending you. Below are some typical reactions.

Appetite: cravings, hunger pangs

Digestion: bloating, constipation, heartburn, gas, cramping, intestinal pain, mucus in stools, diarrhea

Respiratory: stuffy nose or sinuses, postnasal drip, watery or itchy eyes, congestion, persistent cough, sneezing, runny nose

Mood: irritability, anxiety, depression, mood swings

Skin: skin rash, scaly or itchy skin, dark circles under eyes, tongue soreness or cracks, puffy eyes, swelling, acne, rosacea

General/other: water retention, bloating, tiredness, sleepiness, low
energy, insomnia, restless sleep, migraines, headaches, muscle pain,
joint pain, heaviness in limbs, lightheadedness, hot flushes

Sample Journals

To help you see how the reintroduction of foods works, let's take a look
at a real-life example. Remember Leslie, the teacher who was experiencing food reactions, constant bloating, and cravings for cheese and other
dairy products? Here is a page from her journal.

Day	Food	Reactions
Day 1	Yogurt (low-fat), ½ cup	I didn't notice anything.
Day 2	Cheese (low-fat), 1 ounce	I didn't notice anything.
Day 3	Barley, ½ cup	I didn't notice anything.
Day 4	Spaghetti, whole wheat, ½ cup	Felt tired and hungry. Bloating. Heartburn. Mild rash on my face that night.
Day 5	Rye bread, 1 slice	I didn't notice anything.
Day 6	Skim milk, 1 cup	Between breakfast and lunch, I drank 1 cup of milk. I was a bit bloated in the afternoon and had cravings.
Day 7	Bread, whole grain, 1 slice	Heartburn, bloating, cravings. Rash.

Keep a similar journal to record any reactions you may have during the
first week of step 2.

Day	Food	Reactions
Day 1	Yogurt (low-fat), ½ cup	
Day 2	Cheese (low-fat), 1 ounce	
Day 3	Barley, ½ cup	

Day	Food	Reactions
Day 4	Spaghetti, whole wheat, ½ cup	
Day 5	Rye bread, 1 slice	
Day 6	Skim milk, 1 cup	
Day 7	Bread, whole grain, 1 slice	

Here are some tips to help you determine what foods are problematic for you.

- You're going to need to be your own detective and pay close attention to your body. When my clients see me for the first time, some have already suspected that they're sensitive to certain common foods like wheat or dairy and eliminate them *entirely* from their diet. That's not necessary. I don't want to restrict your diet; I just want you to recognize what your boundaries are so you can still enjoy these foods.

- Reactions usually begin to appear one to four hours after you eat a food you don't tolerate, although sometimes they appear the next day. If the food causes symptoms, don't eat it for now.

- If you ate something that aggravated you and it persists, consider taking one Alka-Seltzer Gold tablet with water or ½ to 1 teaspoon of baking soda in water with 500 mg of vitamin C. *Note:* This should not be used by anyone with liver or kidney disease or who is on a potassium-restricted diet. People taking prescription drugs should consult their doctor or pharmacist for advice.

- Do not introduce a new food until any and all reactions from previous foods have subsided.

- Once you've identified your offending foods, you can test smaller amounts to see what your limits are. If you reacted to ½ cup of barley, try ¼ cup. Stay within your boundaries to prevent cravings. The important thing is to get more variety—try not to eat them every day.

- In addition to these foods, people can have intolerances to other foods, although they tend to be less common. For individualized testing, see a health practitioner.

Celiac Disease

Also known as celiac sprue or gluten-sensitive enteropathy, celiac disease is a permanent allergic sensitivity to a protein called gluten, found in wheat, barley, and rye. People with celiac disease often notice pale, malodorous diarrhea accompanied by bloating, gas, and fatigue, but a recent estimate was that 50 percent of people don't experience digestive symptoms but have seemingly unrelated symptoms such as muscle and joint pain.

Undiagnosed celiac disease can be a hidden cause of obesity and is a risk factor for fatty liver. It can also cause nutritional deficiency and weight loss. Most cases of celiac disease are not detected for many years and are finally diagnosed when people are in their thirties and forties. Before they are diagnosed, people are often told they have irritable bowel syndrome.

The prevalence of celiac disease is higher in people of Western European origin. It's typically inherited. Although it was once thought to be rare in the United States, it was recently estimated that as many 1 in 160 people have celiac disease. People with this disease must stay on a gluten-free diet for the rest of their lives or risk causing serious damage to their intestines and nutritional deficiency. Gluten-free foods are buckwheat, amaranth, beans, peas, corn, eggs, millet, potatoes, rice, soy, tapioca, quinoa, and wild rice.

Don't do this test if you have known celiac disease. If you experienced symptoms when you reintroduced rye, barley, or wheat or suspect you may have celiac disease, it's important to get a proper diagnosis. The definitive diagnosis involves a blood test for certain antibodies associated with this disorder.

7

Nourish Your Body to Tame Stress Fat

I don't get angry. I grow a tumor instead.
—FILM DIRECTOR WOODY ALLEN

Chronic stress—whether it's psychological stress or physical stress such as inflammation or pain—promotes the release of the hormone cortisol, causing hunger, elevated blood sugar levels, and fat storage. The Inside Out Diet provides you with the right foods that reduce stress and decrease inflammation. Later, in chapter 11, you'll also learn about lifestyle changes that can help, including mind-body techniques you can do anywhere and tips on improving your sleep.

Cut Back on Caffeine

If you are one of the 80 to 90 percent of adults in North America who drink coffee regularly, I'm not going to recommend you cut out coffee. In fact, coffee has been shown to benefit the liver and, in moderation, lead to a more positive mood and improved performance.

- A study supported by the National Institutes of Health analyzed data on nearly ten thousand people from the National Health and Nutrition Examination Survey. Over two decades, people who consumed the most coffee had the lowest rate of hospitalization or death from liver disease than those who drank little or no coffee. The protective effect was especially so for people with diabetes or people who were overweight.

- Caffeine has been found to improve elevated liver enzymes and prevent acute liver injury by the chemical carbon tetrachloride.

The problem comes when you drink too much caffeine-containing drinks, which can make you dependent on the caffeine and leave you feeling anxious, nervous, irritable, or hypersensitive, and can also cause headaches.

A study at Johns Hopkins University reviewed data from fifty-seven studies and nine surveys on caffeine. It found that addiction can occur with doses of 100 mg and more, and that abstaining from 100 mg or more can cause withdrawal symptoms, which include headache, sleepiness, difficulty concentrating, and irritability. So the key is to have no more than 100 mg a day.

In order to stay within the daily 100 mg caffeine limit, you'll have to check individual brands for the caffeine content. In the last decade, the size and caffeine content of a standard cup of coffee have greatly increased. Gourmet coffees, in particular, often contain double or triple the caffeine. For example, a regular 8-ounce cup of coffee contains about 100 mg. But according to the Nutrition Action Health Letter, an 8-ounce Starbucks coffee has 250 mg of caffeine. Because of supersizing, a "small" can be as much as 12 ounces of coffee and can contain as much as 350 mg of caffeine.

Green Tea

Although most of us are most familiar with black tea, which accounts for 90 percent of all tea sold in North America, it actually comes from the leaves of the same plant, *Camellia sinensis*, as do green tea, white tea, and oolong tea. Tea contains less caffeine than coffee. An 8-ounce cup of black tea, for instance, has between 30 to 50 mg of caffeine, and a cup of green tea has 15 to 40 mg of caffeine, compared with 100 to 350 mg for coffee. Herbal teas, although technically not teas but infusions, usually contain no caffeine.

Flavonoids in green tea called catechins are responsible for many of the health benefits of green tea. One type of catechin, called epigallocatechin-3-gallate (EGCG), is the most widely studied catechin and appears to be the most potent antioxidant of all the green tea catechins. Green tea catechins have been found to:

- Have significantly greater antioxidant activity than vitamin C and vitamin E, in some studies. The antioxidant activity of EGCG is comparable to resveratrol, the antioxidant in red wine that is believed to explain why the French eat one of the richest diets in the world, yet have a lower incidence of heart disease (the "French Paradox").
- Have thermogenic properties, which means they produce heat to burn calories. A study in the *American Journal of Clinical Nutrition* found that people taking a green tea extract increased energy expenditure by 4 percent over twenty-four hours. This is aside from the effects of its caffeine content.
- Detoxify chemicals in the body. Green tea catechins have been found to increase the production of liver enzymes involved in the detoxification of chemicals and protect the liver from damage by toxic substances.
- Reduce liver fat by 55 percent in a study published in the journal *Liver Transplantation*. Catechins are being explored as a treatment for fatty liver in people with liver disease.
- Prevent LDL oxidation, which has been shown to play a key role in the development of arteriosclerosis.
- Prevent cancer. Preliminary studies suggest that EGCG may help to prevent certain cancers.

Green tea also contains a naturally occurring amino acid called L-theanine, which has been demonstrated to enhance brain function, improve concentration, calm and reduce anxiety, and improve mood, without sedation or jitteriness.

The main difference between green and black teas is the way they are processed. Green tea leaves are steamed or pan fired and then rolled and dried, which preserves the EGCG. Black tea leaves are fermented, which results in the deactivation of the majority of catechins. This is why black tea contains about 40 percent of the EGCG in green tea and has a darker color.

Some health practitioners are concerned because green tea contains higher levels of fluoride than black tea, which they see as problematic. However, to put their concern into perspective, green tea has about the same amount of fluoride as a bowl of breakfast cereal.

Although concentrated green tea extracts in pill form may seem like a more convenient alternative to drinking green tea, there have been some reports of liver toxicity after the use of green tea pills. It is not certain that the green tea pills were the cause of the liver problems; however, until we know more, I suggest you avoid the pill form. Also, a 2006 analysis by Consumerlab.com found that some green tea pills were contaminated with lead.

Green tea contains vitamin K, which may decrease the effectiveness of the drug warfarin (Coumadin). If you are taking this medication, speak with your physician before drinking green tea.

There's No Match for Matcha

My favorite type of green tea is matcha. Traditionally the tea of choice used in the Japanese tea ceremony, matcha is also used in cooking, and it adds flavor and color to various foods such as green-tea ice cream. Matcha has a beautiful, vibrant green color, zero calories, and a milder, less bitter taste than other types of green tea.

Matcha is made by grinding green tea leaves to a fine powder after they are dried. The miniscule particles make it easier to extract the catechins when we brew the tea, compared with other types of green tea. The powder is also so fine that it is not strained but is stirred in the cup and consumed.

A University of Colorado study found that matcha has greater potential health effects than other green teas. Specifically, researchers found that matcha had 137 times the amount of EGCG than a popular brand of green tea, and it had three times the amount of EGCG than even the largest reported amount found in any other type of green tea.

Researchers at the Fukuoka Institute of Health and Environmental Sciences found that animals fed matcha excreted up to nine times more PCBs than a control group. They concluded that matcha tea may be a useful treatment for people who are exposed to PCBs and other related chemicals.

How to Make Green Tea

1. Heat filtered water. Remove the water from the heat before it comes to a boil.
2. Use 1 teaspoon of leaves in an infuser or 1 green tea bag. If you are using matcha, use ½ teaspoon of matcha powder. Look for the finest

grind of powder that you can find. You can also strain the entire container of dry tea through a fine sieve to remove larger pieces and then return it to the container afterward.

3. Pour water over the tea leaves. Steep for 1 to 3 minutes.
4. Store the tea in a dry, dark, airtight container. Don't store green tea in the fridge because it can accumulate moisture.

Matcha isn't as easy to find as other types of green tea. Look for it in Japanese grocery stores, tea shops, or on the Internet. If you can't find matcha, enjoy other types of green tea. These tips can help you extract the most EGCG and other catechins during brewing:

- Choose loose-leaf over prebagged tea.
- Compare brands. Younger leaves have a higher EGCG content than mature leaves.
- Look for smaller leaves.
- Steep the leaves for longer than one to three minutes. Although it tastes more bitter the longer it is steeped, more EGCG is extracted. If desired, use a bit of sweetener to take off the bitter edge.

White Tea

White tea is becoming more popular in the United States. Unlike green and black teas that come from the upper leaves of the *Camellia sinensis* plant, white tea comes primarily from the leaf buds, which are covered with silvery hairs that give it a whitish color, and the leaves just under the bud. These buds and leaves are the least processed of all teas. They are lightly steamed and sometimes just dried.

White tea has an amber color and a delicate, subtle taste that many people enjoy. It is slightly sweeter-tasting than many green teas. It also has the least caffeine of the *Camellia sinensis* teas, between 5 and 15 mg per cup. Like green tea, the leaves aren't oxidized, so they are rich in EGCG. White tea appears to have higher levels of EGCG than many types of green tea.

White tea is imported mainly from the Fujian province in China and is only picked once a year, in early spring, which is why it is one of the rarest and most expensive teas. Although I enjoy white tea occasionally, I still prefer matcha. Along with its extremely high EGCG levels, it is one of the most versatile teas (matcha powder can be added to smoothies and other recipes), and is certainly easier on the budget than white tea.

Rooibos Tea

Rooibos (pronounced *roy*-buss) is a caffeine-free reddish brown tea that comes from South Africa. It tastes a lot like regular black tea, except it's less bitter, so many people find that they don't have to sweeten it. Rooibos is rich in the antioxidants called polyphenols, including dihydrochalcones, aspalathin, and nothofagin. Rooibos has been found to improve liver detoxification, boost glutathione levels, and decrease fat in the liver.

Try hot rooibos tea plain, with a wedge of lemon, or with milk. It also makes a great iced tea. Rooibos can also be found mixed with other natural flavors. One of the most popular blends is vanilla rooibos. Spiced rooibos is also good.

Rooibos can be purchased in health food stores, some grocery stores, online, and increasingly, in cafes and restaurants that serve herbal tea. Steep it for about three minutes (unlike regular tea, it doesn't become bitter the longer it's steeped). Some of the more popular brands are Celestial Seasonings, Numi, the Republic of Tea, and Yogi Tea.

Honeybush Tea

If you haven't heard of honeybush tea before, I suggest you look for it and give it a try. Like rooibos, it is from South Africa, but honeybush has a delicious natural sweetness without any calories, which makes it the perfect choice for people who are trying to lose weight. Honeybush tea also has no caffeine. It contains the antioxidants mangiferin, hesperitin, and isokuranetin, and has been found to boost glutathione levels in the liver and improve immune function. Although not yet widely available, honeybush tea can be found in some health food stores, tea shops, and on the Internet.

How to Do It: Have no more than 100 mg of caffeine a day. If you drink coffee, it's important to check individual brands, because caffeine content can vary greatly. Opt for coffee made with water-processed beans, which isn't made with the same chemicals found in processing regular coffee. If you can, also look for blends made from shade-grown coffee beans, which helps to preserve natural forests.

You may wish to try green or white tea. You can also enjoy noncaffeinated teas throughout the day, such as rooibos, honeybush, peppermint, or chamomile teas. During steps 1 and 2, enjoy at least one cup of Cleansing Lemon Tea daily (you can continue to drink it after step 2 if you wish). This easy-to-make tea is designed to help your liver detoxify and reduce gallstones. Lemon peel contains a phytochemical called d-limonene, which gives lemons and other citrus fruits their lemon-orange fragrance. D-limonene aids the liver in neutralizing toxins. Cinnamon protects the liver from excess fat by increasing antioxidants and restoring glutathione.

Consider making time for an afternoon tea break. In traditional tea ceremonies in Asia, the preparation and serving of tea are just as important as actually drinking it. Even if you can spare only five minutes in a busy day, it is still enough time to make yourself a cup of matcha tea, close your office door or retreat into a quiet place, and just enjoy that quiet time for yourself. We carry stress in our bodies and hold it in our minds. Even a few minutes can release stressful thoughts from your mind and make you more able to handle the rest of the day. Buy yourself a beautiful, colorful teacup and create a relaxing afternoon ritual.

Eat Your Veggies

When we are under stress, the inflammatory processes taking place in the body create acidic by-products that can impair the function of our cells, membranes, tissues, enzymes, hormones, and neurotransmitters. This creates a vicious cycle, placing further stress on the body, which worsens inflammation and contributes to weight gain. The Inside Out Diet provides precisely the phytonutrients and antioxidants, in the form of cruciferous vegetables, purple protectors, extraordinary oranges, right whites, and essential fats, that stop the release of anti-inflammatory substances and decrease fat storage.

Further boosting your intake of vegetables—especially raw vegetables—can provide additional help for people who are chronically stressed. Vegetables are rich in antioxidants, and they neutralize the acidic by-products of stress. After they are digested, absorbed, and metabolized, vegetables release bicarbonate into our blood. Fruits, nuts, and root vegetables also do this to a varying degree. Beans and legumes are neutral. At the opposite end of the spectrum, fish, meat, poultry, eggs, shellfish, cheese, milk, and cereal grains release acids into blood that can worsen the metabolic environment if they are eaten too much.

Vegetables also help the sodium-potassium balance in your diet, another key to buffering your body against stress-related health problems. Most of us consume about half as much potassium as we do sodium, because we don't eat enough vegetables and eat too many processed foods that have hidden salt. Stress worsens the problem by causing more potassium to be excreted.

Juicing

Drinking juices from fresh organic vegetables can help you pack more raw vegetables into your diet. There are many benefits to juicing raw vegetables. For example, researchers at Columbia University reviewed medical literature from 1994 to 2003 and found that raw vegetables were more strongly associated with a lower risk of cancer than cooked vegetables. Juicing breaks down the tough plant fibers and concentrates the vitamins, antioxidants, and phytonutrients for immediate absorption, and it stimulates your body to excrete toxins. Vegetable juices also improve the alkaline-acid balance in the body.

As part of the Women's Health Eating and Living Study, researchers at the University of Arizona looked at the impact daily vegetables and vegetable juices had on weight. One group of women in the study was told to eat more fruits and vegetables and drink vegetable juice daily. A comparison group was given weight-loss recommendations but wasn't specifically told to drink juice or eat more vegetables. They found in the first six months a reduction in body weight and body fat in the women drinking the juice, while weight in the other group didn't budge. This study demonstrates how promising vegetables, both whole and in juice form, can be for losing weight and body fat, especially when they are part of a complete program.

The following are some common questions about juicing.

"I'm new at this. What are good vegetables to juice?"

If you're new to juicing, begin slowly. It's best to start with milder-tasting, watery vegetables, such as cucumbers, celery, carrots, fennel, or jicama.

Do not juice cruciferous vegetables, such as spinach, broccoli, or kale. Although one serving a day of raw cruciferous vegetables is acceptable, more than this may impair thyroid function. Cooking deactivates the thyroid-impairing compounds, so try steaming or boiling these vegetables instead.

"Can I store fresh juice in the fridge?"

Fresh juices can be stored in the fridge for up to twenty-four hours, but I suggest you try to drink them within six hours. It's best to store juices in an opaque jar that has an airtight lid.

"Do you recommend buying fresh juice from a store?"

Although making it at home is ideal, many grocery stores are now starting to sell juices made daily. The only problem is that they are often sweet fruit juices, such as orange or grapefruit. Try to find a juice bar that sells pure vegetable juice.

"What kind of juicer should I get?"

If you don't have a juicer already, you can buy a decent one for less than fifty dollars. Of course, there are juicers that run into the hundreds or even thousands of dollars, but if you are just starting out, a basic, inexpensive juicer is all you need right now. In one or two years, if you like, you can upgrade to a premium model, which will extract a greater percentage of juice.

You can make a detoxifying juice blend by mixing the following vegetables in a juicer, after washing them: one small beet, five carrots with the greens removed, two sprigs of parsley, three stalks of celery, and half a cucumber.

Sprouts

When the seeds of vegetables, grains, and beans start growing, they become edible greens called sprouts. Sprouts are fresh, organic raw foods that are an abundant source of antioxidants, vitamins, amino acids, and live enzymes, which makes them easy to digest. Paul Talalay, M.D., from Johns Hopkins University, said in the *American Cancer Society News* that "broccoli sprouts are better for you than full grown broccoli, and contain more sulforaphane, which protects cells and prevents genes from turning into cancer."

Each type of sprout tastes different. Some, like alfalfa or sunflower sprouts, are mild, while others like radish sprouts have a spicy, peppery taste. Sprouts have a delicious texture and flavor when added to salads or enjoyed as a side dish. Prepackaged sprouts are becoming more readily available in supermarkets and health food stores, where they are found in the produce section. They should look moist, crisp, and smell clean with no signs of slime, discoloration, or mold. Sprouts should be stored in the container they came in, or in a loose plastic bag perforated with holes so that water doesn't accumulate. Use them as soon as possible, and don't store them longer than three days.

How to Sprout at Home

If you can't find sprouts at the supermarket or want to save money, try growing sprouts at home. You'll also be ensured the freshest sprouts. Here are some tips and instructions you should know before you get started.

Tips

- Use only certified organic seeds, grains, beans, or legumes meant for consumption. Seeds must be whole (for example, you can't sprout split peas).
- Do not grow sprouts for longer than the recommended length of time.
- You can find sprouting kits online. Some health food stores carry them.
- Great sprouts to try are lentils, clovers, garlic, kale, mustard, broccoli, and buckwheat.
- Don't sprout lima beans, fava beans, tomato, or eggplant seeds, because these can be toxic.
- See the chart on page 107 for detailed instructions on sprouting a variety of vegetables, beans, seeds, and grains.

Instructions

1. Wash your hands thoroughly with soap and water.
2. Get a sterilized jar large enough to hold 4½ to 5 cups.
3. Rinse the seeds thoroughly. Place them in the jar and add filtered water (the water must be from a clean source). You can add liquid grapefruit seed extract (manufacturers recommend twenty drops per gallon of water). Place a cheesecloth or a nylon screen over the opening of the jar and secure it with an elastic band. Soak the seeds for the recommended time.
4. Drain the water with the screen on. Fill the jar again with filtered water to rinse thoroughly. Drain. The seeds must be mostly dry or they will go bad. Place the jar at a 45-degree angle in a drainer to

allow excess water to leave the jar. Seeds should never obstruct the opening or air will not be able to get in.

5. Rinse and drain the sprouts twice a day, once in the morning and once in the evening, for the recommended number of days.

6. On the last day, drain the sprouts completely and store them in a clean, airtight container.

People who are immunocompromised should consult their doctor before eating raw sprouts.

Recommended Sprouting Times

Dry Seeds	Amount	Soaking Time	Sprouting Time	Quantity of Sprouts
Sunflower	1 cup	4 hours	24 hours	2½ cups
Buckwheat	1 cup	15 minutes	24 hours	2 cups
Amaranth	1 cup	3 hours	24 hours	3 cups
Quinoa	1 cup	3 hours	24 hours	3 cups
Lentils	¾ cup	8 hours	3 days	4 cups
Clover	3 tablespoons	5 hours	5 days	4 cups
Garlic	¼ cup	5 hours	5 days	3 cups
Kale	¼ cups	5 hours	5 days	4 cups
Radish	3 tablespoons	6 hours	5 days	4 cups

Part III

The Three-Step Plan

8

Step 1
Jump-Start Your Detox

My doctor told me to stop having intimate dinners for four. Unless there are three other people.

—FILM DIRECTOR AND ACTOR ORSON WELLES

Now that you understand how supporting your liver can help you lose weight safely and permanently, it's time to see your plan come together.

This one-week step has a clear objective: to temporarily remove foods that are congesting your liver and colon and to eat wholesome, healthy foods that support detoxification and decrease inflammation. By doing this, you'll begin to restore insulin and leptin sensitivity, begin burning stored fat, eliminate cravings, reduce fluid and bloating, prevent metabolic slowdown, and ensure healthy weight loss that lasts.

One of the greatest benefits of this one-week step is that when you're ready to begin the next step, you'll introduce one food a day so that you can learn how your body responds to it. It can help you see firsthand how uncontrollable cravings, bloating, and a sluggish system can be related to certain foods.

This diet will launch you into a lifetime of healthy eating. I want you to use this as an opportunity to discover new foods and tastes. A client of mine, an image consultant, told me, "Regardless of how many clothes we have in our closet, most of us wear the same seven outfits, over and over. It's embarrassing, but you've made me realize I cook the same seven meals over and over. My husband and my kids have their favorites— tuna and noodles, spaghetti, macaroni and cheese, fried chicken, and tacos. I hardly ever try anything adventurous, much less these foods here. I can't wait to try these foods, and I'm even going to start fixing something new once a week for my whole family to introduce them to healthier options."

Step 1 at a Glance

This section summarizes the step 1 guidelines of the Inside Out Diet. In order to allow you to customize your plan, some of these foods list only minimums. If you'd like to have two or three colon-cleansing foods a day, for instance, you'll gain further benefit from the detoxifying and satiating effect of these foods.

What to Eat Each Day

- At least 2 servings (1 serving = ½ cup cooked, 1 cup raw, or ¼ cup broccoli sprouts) of cruciferous vegetables
- At least 1 serving (¾ cup) of the purple protectors
- At least 2 servings (1 serving = ½ cup) of the extraordinary oranges
- At least 1 serving of the right whites (¼ cup or 1 garlic clove)
- At least 1 serving of colon-cleansing foods: apples (1 medium or ½ cup applesauce), pears (1 medium), grapefruit (1 small), beans or legumes (½ cup cooked), oats (½ cup cooked), artichokes (1 large or ½ cup artichoke hearts), shirataki noodles (½ cup), carob powder (¼ cup), or fiber powder (1 serving of glucomannan, acacia, guar gum, psyllium, or methylcellulose powders with water)
- As many raw or lightly cooked vegetables as possible
- 1 to 3 servings of lean protein (e.g., 1 scoop whey protein, organic chicken, or turkey)
- 1 to 2 tablespoons ground flaxseeds

What to Drink Each Day

- At least 8 glasses of filtered water
- No more than 100 mg of caffeine a day
- At least 1 cup of Cleansing Lemon Tea (recipe on page 223)

Supplements
- Omega fatty-acid supplement
- Multivitamin

Foods to Enjoy

Poultry (organic, skinless is best)

Chicken

Chicken or turkey sausage
  (preservative free)

Cornish hen

Ground chicken or turkey

Sliced chicken or turkey luncheon meat (preservative free)

Turkey

Turkey bacon (preservative
  free)

Fish (no more than once a week)

Anchovies

Herring

Sardines

Tilapia

Wild salmon (e.g., pink, sockeye, coho, chum)

Protein Powder

Hemp protein   Rice protein   Whey protein

Eggs

Egg whites

Fruits and Vegetables (organic fresh or frozen is best)
Purple Protectors (purple or red in color)

Beets

Blackberries

Black currants

Blueberries

Cherries

Cranberries

Eggplant

Plums

Pomegranate juice, unsweetened

Pomegranates

Purple cabbage

Radicchio

Raspberries

Red apples

Red-purple grapes

Strawberries

Extraordinary Oranges (yellow, orange, or green in color)
Fruits

Apricots

Cantaloupes

Clementines

Guava

Vegetables

Bell peppers
Carrots
Green beans
Leafy greens
Lettuce
Peas, green
Peppers

Pumpkins
Spinach
Squash
Sweet potatoes
Tomatoes
Zucchini

Cruciferous Vegetables

Arugula
Bok choy
Broccoli
Broccolini
Broccoli rabe
Broccoli sprouts
Brussels sprouts
Cabbage (e.g., red, green,
    savoy, napa)
Cauliflower

Chinese cabbage
Collard greens
Kale
Mustard greens
Rutabaga
Swiss chard
Turnip greens
Turnips
Watercress

Right Whites (white or light green in color)

Garlic
Chives
Endives

Leeks
Onions
Scallions

Others

All other fruits and vegetables
Sprouts (e.g., broccoli, sunflow-
    ers, pea shoots, radishes)

Beans and Legumes

All beans and legumes
Miso
Tempeh
Unfermented soy
    (in moderation):

Edamame
Soy milk, low-fat
Soy yogurt
Tofu
Tofu shirataki noodles

Nuts and seeds (raw, unroasted, unsalted preferred; recommended no more than 1 ounce per day)

Almonds

Brazil nuts

Cashews

Chestnuts

Flaxseeds

Hazelnuts

Macadamia nuts

Pecans

Pine nuts

Pistachios

Pumpkin seeds

Sesame seeds

Sunflower seeds

Walnuts

Nut butters made with allowed
  nuts

Healthy Fats and Oils

Almond oil

Avocado

Avocado oil

Dark sesame oil
  (in moderation)

Guacamole

Hazelnut oil

Macadamia nut oil

Olive oil

Olives

Grains and Starchy Carbohydrates

Amaranth

Brown rice (e.g., basmati, jasmine)

Brown rice bread

Buckwheat

100 percent buckwheat
  noodles

Gluten-free bread

Oat bran

Oat groats

Quinoa

Rice noodles

Rolled oats

Sweet potatoes

Wild rice

Beverages

Almond milk, nut milk, oat
  milk, rice milk

Herbal tea, green tea, white tea

Natural coffee substitutes

Organic coffee

Purified water

Raw vegetable juices made
  with allowed vegetables
  (beet or carrot juice,
  maximum 50 percent)

Sparkling water, plain or
  naturally flavored

Condiments, Spices, and Seasonings

Agar flakes
All herbs and spices
Braggs liquid aminos (nonfer-
    mented soy sauce substitute)
Capers
Coconut milk, low-fat
Coconut, shredded, unsweet-
    ened (sparingly)
Herbamare seasoning
Horseradish
Lemon and lime juice
Pure organic extracts (vanilla,
    lemon, almond, etc.)
Salsa
Salt substitute
Sauerkraut
Sea salt
Sea vegetables (dulse, nori,
    kombu, hijiki)
Soy sauce or tamari,
    low-sodium
Tomato paste or sauce
Vinegar (e.g., apple cider,
    balsamic, red wine, rice)

Sweeteners (use sparingly)

Carob powder
Erythritol
Luo han guo
Rapadura, sucanat
Raw yacon syrup
Stevia

Miscellaneous

Greens powder
Lecithin granules

Foods to Eat Rarely

Meat

Beef   Lamb   Pork

Fish and Shellfish

Farmed salmon
Fried or breaded fish
Predatory fish (including bass,
    king mackerel, shark, sword-
    fish, tilefish, tuna, walleye)
Shellfish (including shrimp,
    lobster, mussels, oysters,
    scallops, crab)
Wild chinook or king salmon

Eggs and Dairy

Butter
Cheese
Egg yolks
Milk
Yogurt

Fats and Oils

Hydrogenated, partially hydro-
    genated, or trans fats

Lard

Peanut oil

Vegetable oils (safflower,
    sunflower, soy, corn)

Soy

Soy cheese

Soy ice cream

Soy oil

Soy protein powder

Starchy Foods

Wheat, rye, barley, and millet, and all products made with these
    grains, including bread, pasta, crackers, bagels, cookies, cereal,
    and snack foods (check labels)

Condiments, Spices, and Seasonings

Commercial barbecue sauce
    with sugar

Commercial ketchup with
    sugar

Sauces, seasonings, and spices
    with added sugar

Nuts and Seeds

Peanuts and peanut butter

Sweeteners

Artificial sweeteners (including
    aspartame, sucralose, and
    acesulfame K)

Concentrated fruit sweeteners

Foods containing high-fructose
    corn syrup

Honey

White sugar

Beverages

Alcohol

Sodas

Miscellaneous

Deep-fried foods

Fast food

Keep these tips in mind as you begin:

- Don't allow yourself to go hungry. Saying no to your body when it's sig-
naling you to eat is not healthy and often just triggers overeating. As
your body heals and regains balance, your cravings will subside. But on
the flip side, don't eat when you're not hungry.

- I suggest you avoid dining out as much as possible during the first week of the diet. Because you'll be rather limited in what you can eat, I suggest you start the diet when you will be able to plan for this.

- Eat slowly and chew thoroughly. Digestion of food, especially carbohydrates, starts in the mouth.

- Don't skip breakfast. Eating breakfast gives you sustained energy to carry you through to lunch and also prevents overeating later in the day. If you don't normally eat breakfast or don't feel you have time, try making a smoothie and putting it in a travel mug to have on the way to work.

- Although you don't have to count or measure every bit of food you eat, some people prefer to follow sample menu plans initially to get an idea of the portion size. I've included a sample menu plan for step 1 with approximately 1,500 calories per day, and there are additional menu plans in the appendix for 1,200 and 1,800 calories a day.

   To estimate which menu plan is right for you, multiply your current weight by 10. For example, if you weigh 170 pounds, eating 1,700 calories a day is an approximation of what your body needs to maintain its current weight (although it does not take into account factors like exercise, age, and muscle mass). To lose approximately 1 pound a week, subtract 250 from this number (1,700 − 250 = 1,450 calories, so choose the 1,500-calorie meal plan). To lose 2 pounds a week, subtract 500 calories a week (1,700 − 500 = 1,200, so choose the 1,200-calorie meal plan). If you exercise, you may need to eat more. If the suggested menu plan is not enough food for you, try adding a second snack or increasing portions.

Essential Kitchen Tools

You'll need to stock your kitchen with the following tools and equipment.

- *Glass containers for storing food in the fridge and microwaving.* Avoid storing or microwaving food in plastic containers, plastic wrap, take-out containers, and Styrofoam, which can leave chemical residues in food.
- *Kitchen scissors.* These can be used to quickly chop herbs and other foods. Use them to trim the fat and skin from poultry or to cut meat into smaller pieces.
- *Glass spray bottles to store cooking oil.* Instead of pouring oil from the bottle, the spray bottle allows you to spritz oil onto the pan.

- *Blender or miniblender.* Miniblenders are especially handy because they are smaller and easier to clean.
- *Pans with an enamel finish.* Instead of nonstick pans, try Le Creuset pans that have a matte black interior. These pans haven't been treated with a nonstick coating, and they are easy to clean. You may want to avoid stainless-steel pans for sauteing and frying, because food tends to stick to the surface so you end up using more oil.
- *Measuring spoons.* Metal measuring spoons are convenient. Use them to scoop yogurt directly from the container or to measure berries and vegetables. They're indispensable.
- *Ramekins.* They look like mini soufflé dishes. I have a set from Crate and Barrel and use the smaller (½ cup) size ones for making and serving desserts. You'll know exactly how much you're eating. You can use the larger ones (1 cup) for microwaving breakfast omelets. Just mix the raw ingredients in the ramekin and serve it straight from the microwave.

Meal Plans, Week 1

Capital letters indicate that the recipe is included in this book.

Day 1

Breakfast	Muesli Cereal (use ½ cup blackberries)
Lunch	Maui-terranean Salad with Herbed Chicken and Watercress and Leek Soup
Dinner	Roast Turkey with Roasted Brussels Sprouts, Wild Mushroom Quinoa Dressing, Cranberry Apple Compote, and Cleansing Lemon Tea

Day 2

Breakfast	Asparagus Frittata and 2 slices turkey bacon
Midmorning Snack	Fruit Salad with Orange Mint Dressing
Lunch	Super Green Chicken Soup, salad (1 cup mixed greens, 1 cup arugula, diced red peppers, 1 diced roma tomato) with 1 tablespoon Balsamic Vinaigrette and 1 teaspoon ground flaxseeds
Midafternoon Snack	Cleansing Lemon Tea and apple with 10 almonds

Dinner	4 ounces grilled wild salmon with 1 teaspoon olive oil, 1 cup steamed broccolini, broccoli, or bok choy, with lemon juice and 1 teaspoon olive oil, and ½ cup brown rice mixed with 2 teaspoons ground flaxseeds
Dessert	Carob Mac Nut Drop

Day 3

Breakfast	Blueberry Flax Cereal
Midmorning Snack	apple with 10 almonds and Cleansing Lemon Tea
Lunch	Sweet Potato with Curried Vegetables and Watercress and Leek Soup
Midafternoon Snack	Jicama Sticks with Roasted Red Pepper-White Bean Dip
Dinner	Chicken Stir-Fry over "Rice" and 1 cup steamed spinach or green beans
Dessert	Pomegranate Poached Pear

Day 4

Breakfast	Raspberry Almond Smoothie
Midmorning Snack	apple with 5 almonds and Cleansing Lemon Tea
Lunch	Black-Eyed Pea Stew and 2 teaspoons ground flaxseeds
Dinner	Grilled Chicken Breast with Roasted Vegetable Salsa served on Yellow and Green Zucchini Medley; 1 teaspoon ground flaxseeds

Day 5

Breakfast	Candied Sweet Potato
Midmorning Snack	Pear with 7 walnut halves and Cleansing Lemon Tea
Lunch	Thai Coconut Tempeh and 1 teaspoon ground flaxseeds
Midafternoon Snack	¾ cup blueberries topped with 1 tablespoon sliced almonds

Dinner	Brown Rice and Kale, Vegetarian Chili, and 2 teaspoons ground flaxseeds
Dessert	1 Carob Mac Nut Drop

Day 6

Breakfast	Pumpkin Pie Oatmeal and Cleansing Lemon Tea
Midmorning Snack	½ cup strawberries and ½ cup blueberries topped with 1 tablespoon sliced almonds
Lunch	Chicken Fajita Salad and 1 teaspoon ground flaxseeds
Midafternoon Snack	½ cup Roasted Cauliflower Florets with 5 black olives and 2 tablespoons Chickpea Dip
Dinner	Grilled Turkey Breast Cutlet, Mixed Baby Greens with Blood Oranges, Almonds, and Pomegranates, and ½ cup cooked brown rice with 2 teaspoons ground flaxseeds
Dessert	Lemon Cream with Raspberries

Day 7

Breakfast	2 Southwestern Egg Cups and Cleansing Lemon Tea
Midmorning Snack	½ cup strawberries and ½ cup blueberries topped with 1 tablespoon sliced almonds
Lunch	3 ounces Grilled Chicken Breast, Watercress and Leek Soup, Sweet Potato with Curried Vegetables, and 1 teaspoon ground flaxseeds
Midafternoon Snack	raw vegetables with 2 tablespoons Chickpea Dip
Dinner	Black Bean and Pumpkin Soup with Chicken, Arugula Salad, and 1 teaspoon ground flaxseeds
Dessert	Microwave Apple Crumble

Substitutions

These menu plans are meant to help you come up with ideas. They are not a strict list of meals.

Perhaps you've looked at the menu plan and are not keen on a couple of ingredients. This is your plan, so feel free to try other foods on the list instead and tweak it to suit your preferences and lifestyle. However, if your hesitation concerns a food that is new to you, I encourage you to start slowly and give it a chance. It takes a while to change old habits. For example, when I first started, I really didn't like brown rice. I had grown up eating white rice and bread as my staples, and didn't like the texture or taste of brown rice. But gradually that changed. I learned new recipes and tried different brands and cooking techniques.

Some days, you may be in a particular rush to get out of the house, or perhaps you didn't have a chance to go shopping and don't have the right ingredients on hand. You can substitute these quick and simple options for those in the menu plan. Keep in mind, however, that you'll still have to make sure to meet the daily guidelines (e.g., at least one serving purple protectors, one colon-cleansing food).

Breakfast Options
Blueberry Flax Cereal

Two-Minute Omelet

Snack Options
Small apple or pear with a few almonds

Smoothie

Jicama sticks sprinkled with lime juice and cayenne

2 tablespoons Chickpea Dip with vegetable sticks (e.g., celery, jicama, peeled cucumber, carrots, bell pepper strips, cooked broccoli, roasted cauliflower, belgian endive leaves, cooked asparagus stalks)

Flaxseed Crackers with Salsa

Unsweetened applesauce topped with sliced almonds, toasted flax-seeds, and cinnamon

Lunch Options
3 ounces organic rotisserie chicken (skin removed)

1 cup raw leafy greens (arugula, watercress, radicchio, spinach)

½ cup vegetables (e.g., tomatoes, bell peppers)

Olive oil and balsamic vinegar dressing

Dinner Options

3 ounces skinless chicken or turkey breast

Steamed vegetables: frozen bell peppers, spinach, green beans, green peas, artichoke hearts, snow peas, chopped savoy or napa cabbage, and/or mushrooms

½ cup quinoa or brown rice

Ground flaxseeds

Dessert Option

½ cup berries with 1 teaspoon sliced almonds

Organic Food

A growing body of research is showing that there are more pesticides in our food, environment, and bodies than we previously believed. That is why consumers are willing to pay more to eat organic foods, which are not treated with synthetic chemical pesticides.

If organics are out of your budget or they aren't readily available where you live, here are some tips that can help:

- Buy food in season from local growers. Look for a farmers' market in your neighborhood. There is an online directory of farmer's markets, food co-ops, organic farms, and other local resources at www.localharvest.org.

- Join an organic food-buying club, which is typically a group of seven or more families that buys directly from an organic food distributor. Members are responsible for placing, unloading, and dividing food orders. The Web site www.coopdirectory.org has a list of buying clubs across the country. If you can't find one, consider starting one in your neighborhood.

- If organic food is hard to find where you live, try ordering it online. For example, Fresh Direct delivers in New York and surrounding areas.

- Trim all excess fat from nonorganic meat, poultry, and fish, which is where chemicals accumulate. Choose lower-fat cuts.

- It's worth paying more for organic, especially when it comes to fruits and vegetables that have been found to contain the highest levels of pesticide residues: bell peppers, celery, cucumbers, imported grapes, green beans, leafy greens, pears, potatoes, strawberries, nectarines, peaches, red raspberries, and spinach. The least contaminated foods are avocados, bananas, broccoli, cauliflower, sweet corn, kiwi, mangos, onions, papaya, pineapples, and peas.

- Although pesticide residues are not just in the outer skin but tend to be distributed throughout the fruit/vegetables, you can at least cut down by using either of these methods for washing nonorganic produce with an outer skin (apples, pears, etc.). Do not use these methods for soft, porous fruits and vegetables such as raspberries.

  1. Fill a clean glass basin or sink with cold water until it is half full. Add 1 tablespoon of 35 percent food-grade hydrogen peroxide. Soak fruits and vegetables for five to fifteen minutes depending on how thick or hard the skin is. Drain the water and rinse the produce thoroughly.

  2. Fill a clean glass basin or sink with cold water until it is half full. Add several drops of pure liquid castille soap, which you can find in health food stores in the soap section. Soak fruits and vegetables for five to fifteen minutes and scrub them with a vegetable brush. Drain the water and rinse the produce very well.

What to Expect

In the first few days of step 1, you'll be adjusting to new foods and will be avoiding many foods and chemicals that are rather addictive. Although many people feel energized from day one, in these initial days, it's not uncommon to feel more tired than usual or notice things like gas, irritability, changes in sleeping patterns, acne, headaches, cravings, flulike symptoms, nausea, and body or breath odor. It's important to get as much rest as your body needs, to drink plenty of water, and to not let yourself get hungry. In case you experience increased gas, bloating, or loose stools from eating more fiber and vegetables, cut back slightly and gradually work up to the desired amount.

Keep in mind that if it takes you a few days to feel good, just know that after the initial period, people usually feel better than ever. Of course, if you have any questions or concerns or feel unwell, consult your health-care provider.

The results will be worth it. You'll be rewarded with increased vitality and energy, improved digestion, greater mental focus and concentration, less stress, decreased risk of disease or sickness, and lasting weight loss.

Step 1 Shopping List

This is a shopping list of foods you'll need for the seven-day menu plan here. You may have to visit new grocery stores and health food stores to get some of the ingredients. Refer to the meal plans and recipes for the amounts of the items you will need to buy.

Fruit

Apples
Avocados
Blackberries
Blood oranges
Blueberries
Cranberries, dried
Cranberries, fresh

Cranberry sauce
Fuji apples
Honeydew
Kiwi
Lemons
Limes
Mandarin oranges

Oranges
Pears
Pomegranate seeds
Raspberries
Strawberries

Vegetables

Arugula
Asparagus
Broccoli, brocco-lini, or bok choy
Brussels sprouts
Cabbage
Carrots
Cauliflower
Celery
Collard greens
Garlic
Ginger
Grape tomatoes
Green bell peppers
Jicama

Kale
Leeks
Mixed baby greens
Mixed mushrooms (oyster, shiitake, and cremini)
Mushrooms
Roma tomatoes
Red bell peppers
Red onions
Romaine lettuce
Shallots
Snow pea pods
Spinach or green beans

Sweet white onions (e.g., Maui onion, Walla Walla, Vidalia, Oso)
Sweet potatoes
Swiss chard
Watercress
White onions
Yellow or plain onions
Yellow squash
Zucchini

Poultry and Fish
Boneless, skinless chicken
    breasts, 3 ounces each
Turkey bacon

Turkey breast, 3 ounces each
Wild salmon, 4-ounce pieces

Eggs
Liquid egg whites, small container

Fresh Herbs
Basil leaves   Mint   Thyme
Cilantro leaves   Parsley

Dried Herbs, Spices, Seasonings, and Extracts
Basil   Nutmeg
Bay leaf   Oregano
Cayenne   Pumpkin pie spice
Chili powder   Red pepper flakes
Cinnamon sticks   Smoked chipotle pepper in
Cumin   adobo sauce
Kosher or sea salt   Thyme
Lemon extract   Vanilla extract
Lemongrass

Health Food
Almond milk   Soy yogurt
Carob chips   Stevia
Ground flaxseeds   Tempeh (refrigerated section)
Lecithin   Whey protein, vanilla

Jarred or Canned Goods
Applesauce, unsweetened   Olives
Arrowroot   Olive oil
Balsamic vinegar   Red curry paste
Canned pumpkin   Red wine vinegar
Chicken broth, low-sodium   Rice vinegar
    organic   Roasted red pepper
Coconut milk, low-fat   Soy sauce or tamari,
Diced tomatoes   low-sodium
Green chilies   Vegetable broth, low-sodium
Green curry paste

Nuts and Seeds

Almond butter   Sliced or slivered almonds
Macadamia nuts   Whole almonds
Pecans

Cereal and Grains

Brown rice   Quinoa
Old-fashioned rolled oats

Legumes

Black beans   Hummus
Black-eyed peas   Kidney beans
Garbanzo beans (chickpeas)   White beans

9

Step 2
Ongoing Weight Loss

Eat to live. Don't live to eat.
—MOLIÈRE

You did it! You've reached step 2. Take a moment to appreciate all you've achieved so far: You've begun to normalize the way your body releases sugar and insulin. You've started burning fat. You've decreased inflammation. You've lessened the stress on your body. You've probably noticed that your energy levels are higher than they were before you started the diet—as well as many other improvements in your health, vitality, and appearance. If you're like most people, you may also feel lighter, refreshed, and revitalized. That's a huge accomplishment.

Step 2 at a Glance

Step 2 lasts for three weeks, although many people find this a comfortable step to continue their weight loss until they have reached their desired weight. Begin the first seven days of step 2 by introducing the following foods gradually, using the guidelines in chapter 6 to see if you tolerate them.

- Day 1: Organic yogurt or kefir, low-fat, ½ cup
- Day 2: Cheese (e.g., any type of low-fat cheese), 1 ounce

- Day 3: Barley, ½ cup cooked
- Day 4: Whole wheat spaghetti, ½ cup cooked
- Day 5: Rye bread, 1 slice
- Day 6: Skim milk, 1 cup
- Day 7: Whole grain bread, 1 slice

Only after you've finished checking all of these foods can you can start eating the ones you don't have a sensitivity to on a regular basis. The exception is organic yogurt and kefir. Because of their many health benefits, you can begin eating these two foods after the test day if you don't react to them.

What to Eat Each Day
- At least 2 servings (1 serving = ½ cup cooked, 1 cup raw, or ¼ cup broccoli sprouts) of cruciferous vegetables
- At least 1 serving (¾ cup) of the purple protectors
- At least 2 servings (1 serving = ½ cup) of the extraordinary oranges
- At least 1 serving of the right whites (¼ cup or 1 garlic clove)
- At least 1 serving of colon-cleansing foods: apples (1 medium or ½ cup applesauce), pears (1 medium), grapefruit (1 small), beans or legumes (½ cup cooked), oats (½ cup cooked), artichokes (1 large or ½ cup artichoke hearts), shirataki noodles (½ cup), carob powder (¼ cup), or fiber powder (1 serving glucomannan, acacia, guar gum, psyllium, or methylcellulose powders with water)
- As many raw or lightly cooked vegetables as possible
- 1 to 3 servings lean protein (e.g., 1 scoop whey protein, organic chicken, or turkey)
- At least 1 serving (½ cup) of organic yogurt or kefir, if tolerated, or a probiotic supplement
- 1 to 2 tablespoons of ground flaxseeds

What to Drink Each Day
- At least 8 glasses of filtered water
- At least 1 cup of Cleansing Lemon Tea
- No more than 100 mg of caffeine a day

Supplements
- Omega fatty-acid supplement
- Multivitamin

Foods to Enjoy

Poultry (organic, skinless is best)

Chicken

Chicken or turkey sausage
 (preservative free)

Cornish hen

Ground chicken or turkey

Sliced chicken or turkey breast

luncheon meat (preservative
 free)

Turkey

Turkey bacon (preservative
 free)

Meat (organic/grass-fed preferred; choose lean cuts, trim excess fat)

Beef   Bison   Lamb

Fish (no more than once a week)

Anchovies

Herring

Sardines

Tilapia

Wild salmon (e.g., pink, sockeye, coho, chum)

Protein Powder

Hemp protein   Rice protein   Whey protein

Eggs (omega-3 eggs preferred)

Egg whites

Whole eggs (maximum of 6 each week)

Dairy (organic/low-fat is best; eat only what you can tolerate)

Kefir   Yogurt

Eat only what you can tolerate (once the test period is over)

Low-fat cheeses, sparingly
 (e.g., Swiss, cheddar, parme-
 san, goat)

Low-fat frozen yogurt

Skim milk

Fruits and Vegetables (organic fresh or frozen is best)
Purple Protectors (purple or red in color)

Beets

Blackberries

Black currants

Blueberries

Cherries

Cranberries

Eggplant

Plums

Pomegranate juice, unsweetened

Pomegranates

Purple cabbage
Radicchio
Raspberries

Red apples
Red-purple grapes
Strawberries

Extraordinary Oranges (yellow, orange, or green in color)

Fruits

Apricots
Cantaloupes
Clementines
Guava
Honeydew
Kiwi
Lemons
Nectarines

Oranges
Passionfruit
Peaches
Pears
Persimmons
Pink grapefruit
Tangerines
Watermelon

Vegetables

Bell peppers
Carrots
Green beans
Leafy greens
Lettuce
Peas, green
Peppers

Pumpkins
Spinach
Squash
Sweet potatoes
Tomatoes
Zucchini

Cruciferous Vegetables

Arugula
Bok choy
Broccoli
Broccolini
Broccoli rabe
Broccoli sprouts
Brussels sprouts
Cabbage (e.g., red, green,
   savoy, napa)
Cauliflower

Chinese cabbage
Collard greens
Kale
Mustard greens
Rutabaga
Swiss chard
Turnip greens
Turnips
Watercress

Right Whites (white or light green in color)

Garlic
Chives
Endives

Leeks
Onions
Scallions

Other

All other fruits and vegetables

Sprouts (e.g., broccoli, sunflowers, pea shoots, radishes)

Beans and Legumes

All beans and legumes

Miso

Tempeh

Unfermented soy (in moderation):

Edamame

Soy milk, low-fat

Soy yogurt

Tofu

Tofu shirataki noodles

Nuts and Seeds (raw, unroasted, unsalted preferred; recommended no more than 1 ounce per day)

Almonds

Brazil nuts

Cashews

Chestnuts

Flaxseeds

Hazelnuts

Macadamia nuts

Pecans

Pine nuts

Pistachios

Pumpkin seeds

Sesame seeds

Sunflower seeds

Walnuts

Nut butters made with allowed nuts

Healthy Fats and Oils

Almond oil

Avocado

Avocado oil

Dark sesame oil (in moderation)

Hazelnut oil

Macadamia nut oil

Olive oil

Olives

Omega-3 mayonnaise

Other oils from allowed nuts, seeds, and vegetable oils (in moderation)

Grains and Starchy Carbohydrates

Amaranth

Brown rice (e.g., basmati, jasmine)

Brown rice bread

Buckwheat

100 percent buckwheat noodles

Gluten-free bread

Oat bran

Oat groats

Quinoa

Rice noodles

Rolled oats

Sweet potatoes

Wild rice

Eat only those you can tolerate (once the test period is over)

Barley

Crispbreads (high-fiber, e.g., Wasa, Ryvita)

Rye (rye bread, rye flakes)

Wheat and wheat products (whole wheat pita, whole wheat tortillas, whole wheat pasta, stone-ground whole wheat bread, whole grain, high-fiber bread)

Beverages

Almond milk, nut milks, oat milk, rice milk

Herbal tea, green tea, white tea

Natural coffee substitutes

Organic coffee

Purified water

Raw vegetable juices·made with allowed vegetables (beet or carrot juice, maximum 50 percent)

Sparkling water, plain or naturally flavored

Condiments, Spices, and Seasonings

Agar flakes

All herbs and spices

Braggs liquid aminos (nonfermented soy sauce substitute)

Capers

Coconut milk, low-fat

Coconut, shredded, unsweetened (sparingly)

Herbamare seasoning

Horseradish

Lemon and lime juice

Pure organic extracts (vanilla, lemon, almond, etc.)

Salsa

Salt substitute

Sauerkraut

Sea salt

Sea vegetables (dulse, nori, kombu, hijiki)

Soy sauce or tamari, low-sodium

Tomato paste or sauce

Vinegar (e.g., apple cider, balsamic, red wine, rice)

Sweeteners (use sparingly)

Carob powder

Erythritol

Luo han guo

Rapadura, sucanat

Raw yacon syrup

Stevia

Miscellaneous

Dark chocolate (use sparingly)

Greens powder

Lecithin granules

Foods to Eat Rarely

Meat
Pork

Fish and Shellfish
Farmed salmon

Fried or breaded fish

Predatory fish (including bass, king mackerel, shark, swordfish, tilefish, tuna, walleye)

Shellfish (including shrimp, lobster, mussels, oysters, scallops, crab)

Wild chinook or king salmon

Dairy (avoid any dairy you can't tolerate)
High-fat dairy

Fats and Oils
Hydrogenated, partially hydrogenated, or trans fats

Lard

Peanut oil

Vegetable oils (safflower, sunflower, soy, corn oil)

Soy
Soy cheese

Soy ice cream

Soy oil

Soy protein powder

Starchy Foods (avoid any grains you can't tolerate)
Refined carbohydrates

Condiments, Spices, and Seasonings
Commercial barbecue sauce with sugar

Commercial ketchup with sugar

Sauces, seasonings, and spices with added sugar

Nuts and Seeds
Peanuts and peanut butter

Sweeteners

Artificial sweeteners (including
  aspartame, sucralose, and
  acesulfame K)
Concentrated fruit sweeteners

Foods containing high-fructose
  corn syrup
Honey
White sugar

Beverages

Alcohol

Sodas

Miscellaneous

Deep-fried foods

Fast foods

Meal Plans, Week 2

Capital letters indicate that the recipe is included in this book.

Day 8

Breakfast   Two-Minute Omelet (portions: 3 egg whites, 2
                     tablespoons low-fat coconut milk, and 2 slices
                     turkey bacon)

Midmorning Snack   ½ cup organic low-fat yogurt or kefir (test food)

Lunch   Brussels Sprouts Soup, Grilled Chicken Breast
                     (sliced on 2 cups baby greens with ¾ cup sliced
                     beets, shaved red onion, and diced tomatoes) with
                     1 tablespoon Balsamic Vinaigrette, and 1 teaspoon
                     ground flaxseeds

Midafternoon Snack ½ cup Roasted Cauliflower Florets and 2 table-
                     spoons Hummus

Dinner   Grilled Turkey Breast Cutlet, Mixed Baby Greens
                     with Blood Oranges, Almonds, and Pomegranates,
                     and 2 teaspoons ground flaxseeds

Dessert   Pomegranate Poached Pear and Cleansing Lemon
                     Tea

Day 9

Breakfast   2 Southwestern Egg Cups and 1 teaspoon ground
                     flaxseeds

Midmorning Snack	Cheese (any type of low-fat cheese), 1 ounce (test food)
Lunch	Super Green Chicken Soup, Candied Sweet Potato, and salad (1 cup mixed greens, 1 cup arugula, diced red peppers, and 1 diced roma tomato) with 1 tablespoon Balsamic Vinaigrette
Midafternoon Snack	pear with 7 walnut halves and Cleansing Lemon Tea
Dinner	Chicken Curry, Roasted Cauliflower Florets, steamed spinach, and 2 teaspoons ground flaxseeds
Dessert	¾ cup strawberries

Day 10

Breakfast	Blueberry Flax Cereal with ¾ cup almond milk
Midmorning Snack	Barley, ½ cup cooked (test food)
Lunch	Roasted Vegetable Stew and ¼ cup broccoli sprouts or ½ cup steamed broccoli or broccolini
Midafternoon Snack	Raw vegetables with 2 tablespoons Chickpea Dip
Dinner	Chicken Stir-Fry over "Rice" and steamed green beans or spinach
Dessert	apple with 8 almonds and Cleansing Lemon Tea

Day 11

Breakfast	Two-Minute Omelet (portions: 3 egg whites, 2 tablespoons low-fat coconut milk, and 2 slices turkey bacon) and Cleansing Lemon Tea
Midmorning Snack	Whole wheat spaghetti, ½ cup cooked (test food)
Lunch	Chicken Fajita Salad and 1 teaspoon ground flaxseeds
Midafternoon Snack	raw vegetables and 2 tablespoons Chickpea Dip
Dinner	4 ounces Grilled Chicken Breast, salad (1 cup arugula, 1 cup mixed greens, ¾ cup beets, thinly

sliced red onions, grape tomatoes, 1 tablespoon crushed walnuts, black olives), and 1 tablespoon Balsamic Vinaigrette, 2 teaspoons ground flax-seeds, and ½ cup cooked quinoa

Dessert   1 Carob Mac Nut Drop

Day 12

Breakfast   Raspberry Almond Smoothie

Midmorning Snack   1 slice rye bread (test food)

Lunch   Roasted Vegetable Stew, ½ cup cooked brown rice with 1 teaspoon ground flaxseeds and salad (1 cup mixed greens, 1 cup arugula, diced red peppers, 1 diced roma tomato) with 1 tablespoon Balsamic Vinaigrette

Midafternoon Snack   apple with 12 almonds and Cleansing Lemon Tea

Dinner   Grilled Turkey Breast Cutlet, ½ cup Red Cabbage Live Sauerkraut, steamed spinach, and ½ cup cooked brown rice with 2 teaspoons ground flaxseeds

Day 13

Breakfast   Pumpkin Pie Oatmeal and Cleansing Lemon Tea

Midmorning Snack   1 cup skim milk (test food)

Lunch   Maui-terranean Salad with Herbed Chicken and 2 teaspoons ground flaxseeds

Midafternoon Snack   ½ cup berries and 1 teaspoon toasted ground flaxseeds

Dinner   3 ounces roasted turkey breast, Cranberry Apple Compote, and Arugula Salad

Day 14

Breakfast   Eggs Florentine and 2 turkey breakfast links

Midmorning Snack   1 slice whole grain bread (test food)

Lunch   Chicken Curry, Chopped Salad, and 2 teaspoons ground flaxseeds

Midafternoon Snack	pear slices with 1½ tablespoons almond butter, 1 teaspoon ground flaxseeds, and Cleansing Lemon Tea
Dinner	Chicken Egg Fu Yung with Fried "Rice" and steamed spinach or green beans
Dessert	1 cup berries and ½ cup yogurt

Meal Plans, Week 3

Day 15

Breakfast	Candied Sweet Potato
Midmorning Snack	¾ cup berries, ½ cup low-fat yogurt, 1 tablespoon vanilla protein powder, and 1 teaspoon toasted ground flaxseeds
Lunch	Curried Chicken Salad in Lettuce Wrap, red and green pepper strips, sliced cucumbers, and Cleansing Lemon Tea
Midafternoon Snack	1 cup Roasted Cauliflower Florets with 5 black olives and 2 tablespoons Chickpea Dip
Dinner	Portobello Mushroom with Chicken Cacciatore on Sautéed Swiss Chard and 2 teaspoons ground flaxseeds

Day 16

Breakfast	Cherry Kefir Smoothie
Midmorning Snack	pear
Lunch	Barley-Lentil Soup with Swiss Chard, Chopped Salad, 1 teaspoon ground flaxseeds, and 1 slice bread (e.g., whole grain, rye)
Midafternoon Snack	raw vegetables and 2 tablespoons Chickpea Dip
Dinner	Beef Tenderloin Scaloppini with Puttanesca Sauce and Broccolini, ½ cup cooked barley or quinoa, and 2 teaspoons ground flaxseeds
Dessert	Dark Chocolate Dipped Strawberries

Day 17

Breakfast	¾ cup berries with ¾ cup low-fat yogurt, 2 teaspoons ground flaxseeds, and 2 teaspoons protein powder
Midmorning Snack	1 slice bread with tomato slices drizzled with ½ teaspoon olive oil and balsamic vinegar
Lunch	Brussels Sprout Soup, sliced Grilled Chicken Breast, Italian flat-leaf parsley, thin shavings of parmesan, ½ cup chickpeas, and 1 tablespoon lemon olive oil vinaigrette
Midafternoon Snack	Microwave Apple Crumble
Dinner	Rosemary Grilled Lamb with Goat Cheese, Roasted Beets, Red Onion, and Warm Watercress, 1 teaspoon ground flaxseeds, and Lemon Cleansing Tea

Day 18

Breakfast	Scrambled Egg Oatmeal
Midmorning Snack	pear with 7 walnut halves and Cleansing Lemon Tea
Lunch	Chicken Fajita Salad, ½ cup cooked quinoa, 1 teaspoon ground flaxseeds
Midafternoon Snack	¾ cup blackberries, 1 teaspoon ground flaxseeds, and ½ cup low-fat yogurt
Dinner	wild salmon grilled with 1 teaspoon olive oil, steamed asparagus, ¾ cup artichokes with 1 tablespoon lemon olive oil vinaigrette, and 1 teaspoon ground flaxseeds
Dessert	1 Carob Mac Nut Drop

Day 19

Breakfast	Eggs Florentine and 2 turkey breakfast links
Midmorning Snack	apple with 10 almonds
Lunch	Chicken Egg Fu Yung with Fried "Rice," steamed spinach or green beans, and 1 teaspoon ground flaxseeds

Midafternoon Snack	Jicama Sticks with Roasted Red Pepper-White Bean Dip
Dinner	Grilled Beef Tenderloin Salad and Watercress and Leek Soup
Dessert	½ cup berries, ½ cup low-fat yogurt, and Cleansing Lemon Tea

Day 20

Breakfast	Berry Smoothie
Midmorning Snack	pear with 8 almonds and Cleansing Lemon Tea
Lunch	Curried Chicken Salad in Lettuce Wrap, red and green pepper strips, and sliced cucumbers
Midafternoon Snack	raw vegetables with 2 tablespoons Chickpea Dip
Dinner	Roast Turkey with Roasted Brussels Sprouts, Wild Mushroom Quinoa Dressing, Cranberry Apple Compote, and 2 teaspoons ground flaxseeds

Day 21

Breakfast	Pumpkin Pie Oatmeal
Midafternoon Snack	¾ cup berries, 1 teaspoon ground flaxseeds, and ¾ cup low-fat yogurt or kefir mixed with 2 teaspoons whey protein
Lunch	Eggplant Fresh Mozzarella Salad, 3 ounces sliced Grilled Chicken Breast, and Cleansing Lemon Tea
Midafternoon Snack	pear with 10 walnut halves
Dinner	Lamb Stew and 2 teaspoons ground flaxseeds

Meal Plans, Week 4

Day 22

Breakfast	Blueberry Flax Cereal (use ¾ cup almond milk)
Midmorning Snack	apple
Lunch	Italian-Style Stuffed Red Bell Pepper and Arugula Salad

Midafternoon Snack	Flaxseed Crackers and 1 tablespoon Chickpea Dip
Dinner	3 ounces Grilled Chicken Breast and Brown Rice with Kale and Vegetarian Chili

Day 23

Breakfast	Scrambled Egg Oatmeal
Midmorning Snack	pear with 7 walnut halves
Lunch	Black Bean and Pumpkin Soup with Chicken, 1 slice open-faced bread topped with sliced tomatoes, cheese, and sprouts, and 1 teaspoon ground flaxseeds
Midafternoon Snack	1 cup berries and ½ cup kefir
Dinner	grilled 4-ounce tilapia filet with 2 teaspoons olive oil, ½ cup steamed spinach, ½ cup steamed bok choy or other cruciferous vegetable, ½ cup cooked barley, and 2 teaspoons ground flaxseeds

Day 24

Breakfast	Cherry Kefir Smoothie
Midmorning Snack	apple
Lunch	Black-Eyed Pea Stew and 2 teaspoons ground flaxseeds
Midafternoon Snack	jicama sticks sprinkled with lime juice
Dinner	Grilled Chicken Breast, Roasted Vegetable Salsa, Zucchini Medley, and 1 teaspoon ground flaxseeds

Day 25

Breakfast	Berry Smoothie
Midmorning Snack	apple
Lunch	3 ounces sliced Grilled Chicken Breast, ¾ cup artichokes mixed with 1 tablespoon vinaigrette, ½ cup cooked barley, broccolini, 2 teaspoons ground flaxseeds
Midafternoon Snack	Jicama Sticks with Roasted Red Pepper-White Bean Dip

Dinner	Chicken Cacciatore with Portobello Mushroom and Sautéed Swiss Chard and 1 teaspoon ground flaxseeds

Day 26

Breakfast	2 soft-boiled eggs, 2 turkey breakfast links, tomato slices, and 1 slice bread (e.g., rye)
Midmorning Snack	¾ cup berries with 2 teaspoons ground flaxseeds
Lunch	Barley Lentil Soup with Swiss Chard, Chopped Salad, and 1 teaspoon ground flaxseeds
Dinner	Thai Coconut Tempeh
Dessert	Pomegranate Poached Pear

Day 27

Breakfast	Pumpkin Pie Oatmeal
Midmorning Snack	pear with 10 almonds and Cleansing Lemon Tea
Lunch	Jerusalem Artichoke and Leek Soup, 3 ounces grilled beef or chicken, Arugula Salad with ¾ cup beets, 7 black olives, and 1 tablespoon lemon olive oil vinaigrette, topped with 1 ounce feta or low-fat goat cheese, and 1 teaspoon ground flaxseeds
Midafternoon Snack	2 tablespoons Chickpea Dip with pita wedges (one-half of a 6½-inch-diameter pita) or Flaxseed Crackers
Dinner	Lamb Curry, steamed broccoli, and 2 teaspoons ground flaxseeds

Day 28

Breakfast	Berry Smoothie
Midmorning Snack	1 slice rye bread with tomato slices drizzled with ½ teaspoon olive oil and balsamic vinegar
Lunch	3 ounces sliced Grilled Chicken Breast, ¾ cup artichokes with 1 tablespoon vinaigrette, broccolini, 2 teaspoons ground flaxseeds, and Cleansing Lemon Tea

Dinner	Chicken Stir-fry over "Rice," 1 cup steamed spinach or green beans, and 1 teaspoon ground flaxseeds
Dessert	Microwave Apple Crumble

Healthy Suggestions for Dining Out

If you were able to prepare all your own meals, you would undoubtedly have an easier time avoiding the temptations of other, less healthy foods; this is not always the case, however. Having other people prepare your food (whether at a restaurant, a deli, or any other food establishment) is a fact of modern life, but it doesn't mean your diet has to fall apart because of it. Here are some guidelines to help you stay on track even when eating out.

- Pass on the bread or chips that are brought to your table, or ask the waiter not to bring them at all. Substitute a salad or steamed vegetables instead of pasta, french fries, potatoes, rice, or bread.
- Ask for sauces on the side. For example, request the salad dressing on the side, and choose oil and vinegar instead of creamy dressings.
- Ask for chicken, fish, and seafood to be baked or stir-fried instead of deep-fried.
- Choose dishes that are described as steamed, baked, roasted, poached, broiled, or stir-fried.
- Order plain or sparkling water to drink instead of soda.

Chinese Food

Order chicken or fish with steamed broccoli or other green vegetables as a side dish instead of white rice or noodles. Avoid fried foods, such as spring rolls, chow mein, and fried wontons. Also avoid sweet-and-sour sauces.

Deli Food

Try sliced turkey or chicken breast instead of highly processed meats, and Dijon mustard instead of butter or mayonnaise.

Indian Food

Order tandoori chicken or fish. Bean dishes are other good options. Stick with tomato-based sauces, and stay away from buttery or cream-based sauces.

Italian Food

You can usually order grilled chicken, meat, or fish with a salad. Other options are basil pesto sauce, tomato salad, and chicken marsala. Avoid garlic bread and pasta.

Greek Food

Order grilled chicken, fish, or shrimp and a salad with the dressing on the side.

Japanese Food

Order miso soup, steamed fish, grilled chicken, tofu dishes, and salad. Avoid tempura, which is deep-fried, and teriyaki sauce, which contains sugar. Substitute vegetables for white rice. Enjoy some green tea.

Thai Food

Try fresh spring rolls instead of deep-fried spring rolls, or order soup as an appetizer instead. Avoid fried foods.

Fast Food

In general, I suggest you stay away from fast food because it comes loaded with sugar, salt, and fat. Some of the healthier options are salads or grilled chicken without the sauce. You can try removing the grilled chicken from the bun and eating it with the salad.

10

Step 3
Maintain without Gain

We cannot do everything at once, but we can do something at once.
—CALVIN COOLIDGE

One evening, after our weekly meeting, my client Michelle approached me and said, "I'm a little gun-shy. I don't want to build myself up and then let myself down. Your program fills me with hope, but I'm leery of getting all excited and then losing interest. Any suggestions?" I told her that one of the secrets is not to view this plan as a diet—simply because anything we go "on," we're bound to fall "off." This is a lifestyle.

Step 3 is your lifelong maintenance plan. Five days a week, you'll continue eating the nourishing foods that helped you to lose weight. The other two days are your "flex days." Now that your liver and metabolism are functioning optimally, you can eat moderate amounts of the foods you enjoy, as long as you follow some simple guidelines. You'll continue to feel and look great, without having to "give up" any foods permanently. It will help you maintain your success on The Inside Out Diet.

Step 3 at a Glance

Five consecutive days a week, follow these guidelines each day (the other two days are your flex days):

- Eat at least five servings of colorful fruits and vegetables, including
    Cruciferous vegetables (1 serving = ½ cup cooked, 1 cup raw, or
        ¼ cup broccoli sprouts)
    Purple protectors (1 serving = ¾ cup)
    Extraordinary oranges (1 serving = ½ cup)
    Right whites (1 serving = ¼ cup or 1 garlic clove)
- Eat 1 to 2 tablespoons of ground flaxseeds
- Take an omega fatty-acid supplement
- Drink at least six glasses of water

Flex Days

As I said all along, it was never my intention to create a plan that recommends drastic actions, or that overwhelms or immobilizes you—quite the opposite. Flex days are yet another way The Inside Out Diet helps you stay on track for the rest of your life. Here's how to do it:

- Two consecutive days a week, you may eat whatever you like, unless you are otherwise restricted by food intolerances, heart disease, diabetes, or another health condition. If you like, you may begin your flex days Friday at dinner and end on Sunday at lunch.
- The amount of starchy foods you eat should never be larger than the size of your fist.
- Meat or fish servings should be no larger than the palm of your hand.
- Dessert and sweets should be eaten sparingly. If eating a high-calorie dessert, one serving shouldn't be bigger than a large egg or a golf ball.
- Eat slowly. If you eat quickly, your brain may not have time to register that you're full. Do not overeat or eat when you are not hungry.
- Avoid fast food, deep-fried food, sugary food, or junk food.

Foods to Enjoy

Poultry (organic, skinless is best)

Chicken

Chicken or turkey sausage
   (preservative free)

Cornish hen (preservative free)

Ground chicken or turkey

Sliced chicken or turkey breast
   luncheon meat (preservative
   free)

Turkey

Turkey bacon (preservative free)

Meat (organic/grass-fed preferred; choose lean cuts, trim excess fat)

Beef	Bison	Lamb

Fish (no more than once a week)

Anchovies	Tilapia
Herring	Wild salmon (e.g., pink, sock-
Sardines	eye, coho, chum)

Protein Powder

Hemp protein	Rice protein	Whey protein

Eggs (omega-3 eggs preferred)

Egg whites
Whole eggs (maximum of 6 each week)

Dairy (Organic/low-fat is best; eat only dairy you can tolerate)

Kefir	Low-fat frozen yogurt
Low-fat cheeses sparingly	Skim milk
(e.g., Swiss, cheddar,	Yogurt
parmesan, goat)	

Fruits and Vegetables (organic fresh or frozen is best)
Purple Protectors (purple or red in color)

Beets	Pomegranate juice, unsweetened
Blackberries	Pomegranates
Black currants	Purple cabbage
Blueberries	Radicchio
Cherries	Raspberries
Cranberries	Red apples
Eggplant	Red-purple grapes
Plums	Strawberries

Extraordinary Oranges (yellow, orange, or green in color
Fruits

Apricots	Kiwi
Cantaloupes	Lemons
Clementines	Nectarines
Guava	Oranges
Honeydew	Passionfruit

Peaches

Pears

Persimmons

Pink grapefruit

Tangerines

Watermelon

Vegetables

Bell peppers

Carrots

Green beans

Leafy greens

Lettuce

Peas, green

Peppers

Pumpkins

Spinach

Squash

Sweet potatoes

Tomatoes

Zucchini

Cruciferous Vegetables

Arugula

Bok choy

Broccoli

Broccolini

Broccoli rabe

Broccoli sprouts

Brussels sprouts

Cabbage (e.g., red, green,
   savoy, napa)

Cauliflower

Chinese cabbage

Collard greens

Kale

Mustard greens

Rutabaga

Swiss chard

Turnip greens

Turnips

Watercress

Right Whites (white or light gree in color)

Garlic

Chives

Endives

Leeks

Onions

Scallions

Other

All other fruits and vegetables

Sprouts (e.g., broccoli,

sunflower, pea shoots,

radishes

Beans and Legumes

All beans and legumes

Miso

Tempeh

Unfermented soy
   (in moderation):

Edamame

Soy milk, low-fat

Soy yogurt

Tofu

Tofu shirataki noodles

Nuts and Seeds (raw, unroasted, unsalted preferred; no peanuts; recommended no more than 1 ounce per day)

Almonds

Brazil nuts

Cashews

Chestnuts

Flaxseeds

Hazelnuts

Macadamia nuts

Pecans

Pine nuts

Pistachios

Pumpkin seeds

Sesame seeds

Sunflower seeds

Walnuts

Nut butters made with allowed nuts

Healthy Fats and Oils

Almond oil

Avocado

Avocado oil

Dark sesame oil (in moderation)

Hazelnut oil

Macadamia nut oil

Olive oil

Olives

Omega-3 mayonnaise

Organic butter (sparingly)

Other oils from allowed nuts, seeds, and vegetables (in moderation)

Grains and Starchy Carbohydrates

Amaranth

Brown rice (e.g., basmati, jasmine)

Brown rice bread

Buckwheat

Gluten-free bread

100 percent buckwheat noodles

Oat bran

Oat groats

Quinoa

Rice noodles

Rolled oats

Sweet potatoes

Wild rice

Eat only those you can tolerate

Barley

Crispbreads (high fiber, e.g., Wasa, Ryvita)

Rye (rye bread, rye flakes)

Wheat and wheat products

(whole wheat pita, whole wheat tortillas, whole wheat pasta, stone-ground whole wheat bread, whole grain, high-fiber bread)

Beverages

Almond milk, nut milk, oat
  milk, rice milk
Herbal tea, green tea,
  white tea
Natural coffee substitutes
Organic coffee
Purified water

Raw vegetable juices made
  with allowed vegetables
  (beet or carrot juice,
  maximum 50 percent)
Red wine (sparingly)
Sparkling water, plain or
  naturally flavored

Condiments, Spices, and Seasonings

Agar flakes
All herbs and spices
Braggs liquid aminos
  (nonfermented soy sauce
  substitute)
Capers
Coconut milk, low-fat
Coconut, shredded,
  unsweetened (sparingly)
Herbamare seasoning
Horseradish
Lemon and lime juice
Pure organic extracts (vanilla,
  lemon, almond, etc.)

Salsa
Salt substitute
Sauerkraut
Sea salt
Sea vegetables (dulse, nori,
  kombu, hijiki)
Soy sauce or tamari,
  low-sodium
Tomato paste or sauce
Vinegar (e.g., apple cider,
  balsamic, red wine, rice)

Sweeteners (use sparingly)

Carob powder
Erythritol
Luo han guo

Rapadura, sucanat
Raw yacon syrup
Stevia

Miscellaneous

Dark chocolate (use sparingly)
Greens powder

Lecithin granules

Foods to Eat Rarely

Meat

Pork

Fish and Shellfish

Farmed salmon

Fried or breaded fish

Predatory fish (including bass, king mackerel, shark, swordfish, tilefish, tuna, walleye)

Shellfish (including shrimp, lobster, mussels, oysters, scallops, crab)

Wild chinook or king salmon

Dairy (avoid any dairy you can't tolerate)

Butter

High-fat dairy

Fats and Oils

Hydrogenated, partially hydrogenated, or trans fats

Lard

Peanut oil

Vegetable oils (safflower, sunflower, soy, corn)

Soy

Soy cheese

Soy ice cream

Soy oil

Soy protein powder

Starchy Foods (avoid any grains you can't tolerate)

Refined carbohydrates

Condiments, Spices, and Seasonings

Commercial barbecue sauce with sugar

Commercial ketchup with sugar

Sauces, seasonings, and spices with added sugar

Nuts and Seeds

Peanuts and peanut butter

Sweeteners

Artificial sweeteners (including aspartame, sucralose, and acesulfame K)

Concentrated fruit sweeteners

Foods containing high-fructose corn syrup

Honey

White sugar

Beverages

Sodas

Miscellaneous

Deep-fried foods

Fast food

Typical Portion Sizes

Fist = 1 cup

Thumb from tip to closest knuckle = 1 tablespoon

Dice = 1 teaspoon

Golf ball or large egg = ¼ cup

Thumb = 1 ounce

Deck of cards = 3 ounces

11

Daily Essentials

Exercise, Relaxation, Sleep, Healthy Home, and Journaling

Thank you for calling the weight-loss hotline. If you'd like to lose half a pound right now, press 1 eighteen thousand times.

—CARTOONIST RANDY GLASBERGEN

Are you tired of forcing yourself to exercise or feeling guilty because you don't? Join the club. Regular exercise is one of the leading predictors of long-term weight loss—and one of the hardest things to stick to. But it's worth it.

The Importance of Getting Enough Exercise

Combined with dieting, exercise increases your weigh-loss capacity by helping you burn calories, and it can make a greater impact on the health of your liver than diet alone. Exercise also has the following benefits:

- Increases energy and stamina
- Improves insulin sensitivity and can lower blood sugar
- Strengthens the cardiovascular system, reducing the risk of heart disease, stroke, and high blood pressure
- Aids digestion
- Reduces hunger

- Improves mood by activating neurotransmitters and endorphins
- Builds muscle
- Preserves bone mass, keeping bones strong
- Reduces the risk of certain types of cancers
- Strengthens the immune system
- Improves sleep
- Prolongs life span

That's why it's worth developing a workout plan you can stick to. Other daily essentials that keep you healthy and detoxify are getting adequate sleep, keeping your home healthy, skin brushing, learning mind-body relaxation techniques, and keeping a journal.

Make Thirty Minutes a Day Your Target to Start

In order to reap the benefits of exercise, you'll need to exercise at least thirty minutes a day. Although this may seem like a lot, you don't have to do it solely by putting in time at the gym. What often works is four days a week of structured exercise and then three days a week of anything that gets you moving, whether it's dancing, golfing, or raking leaves, as long as you do it with enough intensity.

Aerobic Exercise

Aerobic exercise, in which the heart and lungs must work harder to meet increased oxygen demands, is part of a complete exercise plan, which should also include resistance training and flexibility exercises. When we think aerobics, many of us think of the treadmill, Stairmaster, or, God forbid, the dated eighties' workout trend. But there are actually many options to get the heart pumping (and none of them require leg warmers and headbands).

Brisk Walking

Walking is an excellent form of exercise, especially when you are just beginning an exercise plan or haven't exercised in a while. Regular, brisk walking can help you lose fat if you walk quickly and frequently. Brisk walking means walking as if you might be late for a meeting or miss a bus. It also doesn't cost anything or require any special equipment, which is why it is easy to stick with.

Many studies have found that walking can also improve risk factors of chronic disease and boost mood. A study by researchers at Dalhousie

University, in Halifax, Nova Scotia, found that thirty-minute walks were effective at reducing tension, anxiety, and mood disturbance and increasing energy and vigor. My clients who start incorporating brisk walking into their day notice an improvement in energy, concentration, and mood.

I enjoy taking walks first thing in the morning, when the air is crisp and the streets are quiet. Outdoor walking gives you the time to reflect and gain perspective. You can even combine walking with daily errands, rather than drive, which makes it less likely that you'll cut your workout short. Just remember to start slowly, increasing the length and intensity gradually.

If you walk regularly, you may wish to get a pedometer or a step counter to keep track of how much you are walking a day. It can help motivate you. A company called Omron makes a pedometer that you can conveniently put in your pocket or purse, or clip it to your belt, rather than strap onto your ankle. If you are walking to lose weight, strive for 10,000 to 12,000 steps a day. To put it in perspective, routine activities throughout the day equal about 4,000 steps and walking one mile equals about 2,000 steps.

Measuring Your Heart Rate

Gently place your index finger of one hand on the radial artery, which is on the underside of the opposite wrist at the end, closer to the thumb. Count the beats for a full sixty seconds. You can also try counting beats for fifteen seconds and multiplying the number of beats by four. Just be consistent and keep in mind that the longer you count, the more accurate the result.

Here's how to calculate your maximum heart rate. Your maximum heart rate is 220 minus your age. For example, the maximum heart rate for a thirty-five-year-old is 185 (220 − 35 = 185). Multiply your maximum heart rate by 0.6. This is the minimum your heart rate should be during exercise. So, based on our earlier example, the minimum heart rate for a thirty-five-year-old is 111 (185 × 0.6 = 111).

If you are going to walk regularly, consider investing in a heart-rate monitor to calculate your heart rate. A typical heart-rate monitor costs about eighty dollars and includes a strap that you place around your chest and a monitor that is usually also a wristwatch. Heart-rate monitors can interfere with pacemakers or other implanted devices, so read the manufacturer's specifications and consult your doctor if in doubt.

Jumping Rope

Jumping rope is another convenient and effective option. It promotes fat loss; improves circulation; maintains and improves bone density; helps with balance and coordination; works your major muscle groups, including your thighs, arms, glutes, shoulders, chest, and abdomen; and burns plenty of calories.

Jumping rope may help prevent the formation of cellulite, by improving the flow of blood and lymph. One of the factors contributing to the development of cellulite is poor circulation to connective tissue—the network of fibers underneath the skin—which causes swelling that can then stretch connective tissue and cause fat to protrude.

The following tips will make your rope jumping more effective.

- Choose a jump rope made of plastic. Cloth ropes tend to be flimsy and light. Make sure it's the right length. Stand on the center of the rope and pull the ends straight up alongside your body. The handles should reach your armpits on both sides.
- Start slowly. Begin with sets of two to three minutes, followed by brisk walking in place or strength-training exercises. Gradually increase the number and length of sets.
- Don't try to move your upper body or arms too much when you skip. Keep your shoulders down and back and elbows close to your sides, allowing most of the movement to come from your wrists. Feet should be about shoulder-width apart.
- Don't try to jump too high; just high enough to clear the rope is fine. Land softly on the balls of your feet (aerobics or cross-training shoes are best because they have better forefoot padding than running shoes). Avoid concrete floors.
- Warm up and cool down for ten minutes each by walking in place and doing some light stretching.
- *Note*: People with high blood pressure, osteoporosis, or arthritis shouldn't try jumping rope unless they have consulted with their doctor.

Resistance Training

Resistance exercises, such as lifting weights or using resistance bands and balls, are another key component of your exercise plan. Toned muscles have more insulin receptors, which means more sugar is burned as fuel rather than stored as fat.

Strength training may also prevent stress-fat from accumulating in the abdomen. For example, a study in the *Journal of Applied Physiology* divided women into four groups: one group followed a diet; another group dieted and did aerobics; the third, a combination of diet, aerobics, and strength training; and the fourth did nothing. The researchers found that cortisol levels measured at the end of the study had risen by 51 percent in the diet and aerobics group compared to a much smaller rise of 10 percent in the group that combined diet, aerobics, and strength training. Bottom line: strength training controls cortisol more effectively when combined with aerobics than aerobics alone.

If you have never lifted weights before or have a history of injuries, it would be wise to work out with a trainer, at least initially, to ensure that you are using proper technique, pushing yourself hard enough, and are not putting yourself at risk for injury.

What Works Best for *You*?

One of my clients insisted she was a klutz and hated all sports. She said, "I grew up in a family of brothers. They played games with the neighborhood kids on our street morning, noon, and night. Anytime I tried to join in, they'd laugh at my awkwardness and make jokes because I couldn't hit, catch, or throw the ball. I guess I let them get to me because I'm still afraid to try any new types of exercise."

Have past experiences formed habitual attitudes and behaviors that undermine your health? Do you agree with Joan Rivers, who said, "I don't exercise? If God wanted me to bend over, he would have put diamonds on the floor?"

It may be time to look those obstacles in the eye and find something you can enjoy—and stick to. Take a moment to think about your preferences and lifestyle. These questions will help give you some ideas.

- When do you most enjoy exercising? What's the most convenient time for you?
- What current scheduling factors help or hinder your ability to engage in a workout program? Work? School? Day care?
- Do you like going to the gym? Why or why not?
- Do you like exercising by yourself or with friends?
- Have you had problems keeping up your motivation to work out?

Choose a Consistent Time to Work Out

Although routines can be boring, a proven strategy that can really help you stick with your plan is to maintain a regular workout schedule. Exercise around the same time every day, whether it's in the morning, during a midafternoon break, or in the evening. Right after work may be the most convenient for you. Or, you may find that working out first thing in the morning makes you more productive during the day. If you are at home with the kids, midmorning might be the best time for you. A consistent schedule will make it as much of a priority as brushing your teeth.

Make Sure It's Convenient

If it takes you more than half an hour to get to the gym, you might find yourself skipping exercise because you just don't have the time. Look for a gym that is close to home or work. If there isn't one, it may mean exercising outdoors, by going for an hour-long walk in the evening. Or, you can buy home exercise equipment and workout DVDs and set up a small home gym. Although it requires more of an investment initially, there are no membership fees (which can add up), you may be more likely to exercise regularly, and it can save traveling time.

You Don't Have to Do It All at Once

Getting your daily exercise is not an all-or-nothing deal. Exercising in short bouts throughout the day is just as helpful as doing it all at once, especially if it means you're more likely to stick with it. Also, it gives people who would otherwise be snacking something to do. So even if it's ten-minute sessions—it all adds up!

Mix It Up

Adding variety to your workouts not only makes it more interesting, it decreases the risk of injury. Try alternating your regular workout with activities like walking, dancing, tennis, going on a bike ride, or skating.

Start Slowly

Although it is tempting to jump right in to a new exercise routine, it's important to start slowly and gradually increase the length and intensity of your exercise.

Before starting an exercise program, consult your doctor and have a complete checkup, especially if you are over fifty or haven't exercised regularly in six months. If you have or are at risk for heart disease, diabetes, osteoporosis, or other conditions, get your doctor's approval first.

Enhance Your Circulation

Gentle skin brushing can facilitate detoxification by improving blood and lymph flow and removing dead skin cells, allowing some fat-soluble toxins to be excreted through the skin. In addition to detoxification, skin brushing keeps skin looking youthful and may even slow the development of cellulite. It stimulates circulation, bringing antioxidants, water, and nutrients to the skin. Skin brushing also exfoliates by stimulating the turnover of skin cells. It takes only a few minutes and feels great before a shower.

Here's how to brush your skin.

1. Use a long-handled natural bristle brush. Look for one at a health food store. If you are unable to find one, use a loofah sponge.
2. Start at your feet. Using light pressure, brush in small circles from the feet, up the legs toward the chest, then the palms of the hands toward the chest, and then the back toward the abdomen.
3. Avoid the face, breasts, and other sensitive areas. Don't apply too much pressure or cause redness or irritation. Skin brushing can be done in the morning or evening by itself or before a shower.

Get Serious about Stress Reduction

Mind-body techniques are proving to be effective in controlling appetite and helping with weight loss.

Relaxation Techniques

Progressive muscle relaxation is a technique that involves tensing and relaxing each muscle group in the body, starting from one end, usually the feet, and working toward the other. A pilot study at the Medical University of South Carolina looked at twenty minutes a day of progressive muscle relaxation compared to twenty minutes of quiet sitting. After eight days, people who used progressive muscle relaxation had a significant reduction in stress, fatigue, anxiety, depression, and cortisol levels. They also ate more at breakfast and were less vulnerable to nighttime cravings and eating.

Yoga combines postures, breathing, and meditation. It can help to improve strength and flexibility. An analysis of the data from the Vitamin and Lifestyle (VITAL) study, involving 15,550 adults, found that yoga practice for four or more years was associated with 18.5 pounds less weight gain compared with people who didn't practice yoga.

Meditation can involve concentrating on a specific word or mantra, or it can involve increasing awareness, such as in mindfulness meditation. In one study, 140 people with binge eating disorder practiced mindfulness meditation or were put on a waiting list for counseling. At the end of the study, people in the mindfulness group had significantly fewer binge days per month and improved glucose and insulin responses to food than the people on the waiting list.

Two-Minute Relaxation

One of the most simple yet effective tools to relax is the following breathing technique, which has a powerful physiological effect on the body, helping to calm and destress you in short order while simultaneously restoring your energy and stamina. It also enhances circulation, relaxes muscles, decreases heart rate, and helps you detoxify and improve your metabolism.

1. *Adjust your posture.* Sit in a chair with your feet on the floor and your arms resting lightly on your thighs. Sit up straight with your shoulders down and back. If you can, loosen any restrictive clothing, particularly around the waist. Identify any areas of tension in your body and consciously relax them.

2. *Become aware of your breathing.* Inhale gently through your nose. Your inhalation shouldn't be forceful, and it shouldn't make your head move. It should be slow and steady. Don't hold your breath.

   Exhale through your mouth. Again, this should be slow and even. Your lips shouldn't be pursed or tensed but soft and relaxed.

3. *Use your diaphragm to breathe.* Many people hold in their abdomen out of habit, sit at the computer hunched over, or wear clothing that is tight around the waist. All of these things contribute to shallow, restricted breathing that is confined to the upper chest area.

   Proper breathing involves the diaphragm, a sheet of muscle at the base of the chest cavity, beneath our lungs, and our primary muscle for breathing. When it contracts, it allows our lungs to fill with air. When we don't use our diaphragm or breathe shallowly, our lungs don't completely fill, making us tired, anxious, and tense.

Place one hand flat on your abdomen just below your ribs. Now inhale and release the belly so that it expands outward as it fills with air. Think of your abdomen as being soft and expandable.

Gradually exhale. Your hand should slowly return to the starting position.

4. *Count your breaths.* The final step is to inhale as you mentally count slowly, starting from one. When people are starting out, they can typically inhale for a count of three.

Double this number; that is how long an exhalation should last. If you counted to three when you inhaled, count to six when you exhale. You'll find with practice that your breaths naturally become longer.

That's it! Now repeat it four or five more times. As you practice, you will become more effective at relaxing yourself, letting go of your thoughts, and focusing on your body and the moment.

Become a Mindful Eater

When was the last time you sat down at a table and had a meal without reading, watching television, or thinking about what you had to do afterward? A pilot study at Indiana State University found that mindfulness training, including specific instructions to slowly savor food and be aware of how much food is enough, helped to reduce eating binges from an average of four binges per week to one and a half.

By slowing down the pace of your eating, research shows you can save approximately sixty-seven calories per meal. If you do that for two meals a day, that's fourteen pounds by the end of the year!

How to Do It: Instead of scarfing down your food so quickly you don't even realize you're full, become a mindful eater.

Eliminate all distractions, and savor, rather than inhale, your food. Slow down the pace of your eating.

Pay full attention to what the food looks like on your plate, how it smells, and how it tastes. Chew slowly. Be aware of how full you are becoming. Use a three-point scale: 0 is hungry and 3 is stuffed; aim for 2, which is content. People often notice that food tastes better this way and is more filling. It's as simple as that.

Get Enough Sleep

Lack of sleep may be keeping you from losing weight. A Columbia University study examined data from a large sample of people in the United States over the course of ten years. They found that the people who slept less than seven hours a night had higher body mass indexes and were more likely to be obese than people who slept more than seven hours a night.

Sleep loss appears to cause hormonal changes that promote weight gain. Researchers at the University of Bristol demonstrated that people who slept for five hours a night had 15 percent more ghrelin, a hunger-promoting hormone. These people were also found to have 15 percent less leptin, a hormone that naturally suppresses appetite. Other studies have found that when sleep is cut short, people tend to eat more sweet and starchy foods. Loss of sleep disturbs glucose metabolism and insulin sensitivity, which can also lead to hunger and weight gain.

Here are some tips for improving your sleep.

- Sleep in a dark room. Make sure the temperature of the room is neither too hot nor too cool. According to the Better Sleep Council, between 60 and 65 degrees Fahrenheit is ideal.
- Sip a cup of chamomile tea one to two hours before bed. *Note*: Chamomile may increase the risk of bleeding if used in combination with anticoagulant medications such as Coumadin (warfarin), heparin, Plavix (clopidogrel), Ticlid (ticlopidine), or Trental (pentoxifylline). Consult your doctor if you are taking these medications.
- Avoid big meals within three hours of going to bed. Digestion requires energy and may keep you up.
- Set a regular bedtime. Allow yourself some time to unwind beforehand. For example, if 10:30 p.m. is your bedtime, relax or read from 10 to 10:30 p.m.
- Try putting a drop of scented essential oil in some body lotion and massaging it into your neck or temples.
- Avoid coffee, alcohol, and other stimulants before bedtime because they can interfere with sleep.
- Make your bedroom a restful haven. Splurge on good pillows. Also consider treating yourself to soft sheets with a thread count of at least three hundred. If your bedroom is cluttered or full of work, try clearing it and removing anything that could distract or upset you.

- Don't eat refined, processed carbs, especially in the evening, because they can cause blood sugar fluctuations and wake you up in the middle of the night.
- Regular exercise can improve your ability to fall asleep.
- Avoid using sleeping pills. Consider consulting an herbalist about herbal sleep remedies such as valerian, which has been found to improve the duration and quality of sleep. Valerian is not recommended as a long-term sleep remedy, however.

Make Your Home Healthier

Up to now, I've focused on the chemicals in food and water. But the air we breathe is also a considerable source of chemicals. Airborne pollutants can enter our water supply through emissions and runoff and wind up in our bodies. According to the Environmental Protection Agency (EPA), there are as many as eight hundred volatile organic chemicals wafting in our indoor air, where we spend 90 percent of our time. They are not just found in furniture, computers, cleaners, or carpets that give off a strong or "new" scent. Whether you're able to smell them or not, our homes contain so many chemicals, such as formaldehyde, trichloroethylene, and benzene, that the EPA ranks indoor air pollution one of the top five environmental risks to our health. Following are some of the most simple and effective ways you can remove these chemicals.

Eliminate Environmental Toxins and Other Hazards

Reducing the amount of chemicals in your home and office is the logical first step. The following tips can help make your home cleaner and healthier.

- Avoid using chemical air fresheners and deodorizers. Open a window instead for ventilation. The air inside our homes contains two to five times the pollution of outdoor air. Or try placing an open box of baking soda near odors to absorb them.
- Use natural cleaners instead of chemical ones. You can find natural cleaners at health food stores. You can also make your own. For example, combining a quarter cup of baking soda with just enough water to form a toothpastelike consistency can be used instead of abrasive commercial cleaners. Another great natural cleaner is vinegar.

- Wash bed sheets in the washing machine using hot water two to four times a month.

- Use nontoxic laundry detergent and dish detergent, which you can find in health food stores and natural grocers. Don't use chlorine bleach.

- Don't buy stain-repellent fabrics.

- When purchasing upholstered furniture, computers, and mattresses, ensure that they haven't been treated with the fire-retardant polybromi-nated diphenyl ether (PBDE). North Americans have the highest PBDE levels in the world. PBDE has been linked in animal studies to thyroid and reproductive disorders and immune system suppression. Once in the body, it's believed to break down into estrogenlike com-pounds. Many companies have already phased out PBDE. Contact individual manufacturers for information.

- Dust and dryer lint are full of chemicals. A study by the National Insti-tute of Standards and Technology examined house dust and dryer lint in a sample of Washington, D.C., area homes and found PBDE in all samples. Keep dust levels low with regular cleaning. Invest in a good vacuum cleaner or a central vacuum system. Avoid bagless vacuum cleaners, which can release dust into the air when you are emptying the bin. Be careful when removing dryer lint from your dryer and always wash your hands afterward.

- Consider getting an air filter. The best type of air filter is one that uses HEPA and activated carbon. HEPA, which stands for high-efficiency particulate air, is a technology that was first developed in the 1940s by the United States Atomic Energy Commission to remove radioactive plutonium particles inside its labs. With HEPA filters, a fan pulls air through foam to filter out the larger particles. Air then enters the HEPA filter, which removes microscopic particles. The most efficient HEPA filters remove 99.97 percent of particles down to a size of 0.3 micron. HEPA filters are not as helpful as other filters in removing airborne chemicals, however.

  Activated carbon filters are carbon filters that are treated with steam to increase the number of microscopic pits, which physically trap airborne particles. What makes these filters unique is that, unlike HEPA filters, they also soak up chemical gases by a process called adsorption and are better at reducing odors.

- Explore alternatives to conventional dry cleaning. It's estimated that 85 percent of dry cleaners use a chemical solvent called perchloroethylene, or perc, which ends up in our air, ground, and water. Three alternatives are GreenEarth, a silicone-based solvent; liquid carbon dioxide; or "wet cleaning," which uses plain water. Consumer Reports found that the carbon dioxide and silicone-based solvents do a better job at preserving fabric than conventional dry cleaning. Many people consider wet cleaning to be the safest and most cost-effective method, but it may not be the best choice for wool.

Improve the Quality of Your Air with Houseplants

A little-known, inexpensive way to remove potentially toxic chemicals from the air is with houseplants. Bill Wolverton, Ph.D., a former NASA research scientist and the author of *How to Grow Fresh Air*, pioneered the use of house and office plants to reduce indoor air pollution. Plants literally soak up chemicals and can even break them down. Houseplants also naturally moisturize the surrounding air. For most living areas, one to two potted plants per 100 square feet is adequate, although in some areas, such as around new furniture and computers, three plants are ideal.

Indoor Palms

Palms make striking indoor plants. Many of them have large leaves with bold shapes. Three indoor palms that have been found to filter chemicals from the air are:

1. *Bamboo palm*. A tall, narrow plant with clusters of long, slender leaves.
2. *Areca palm*. A popular indoor palm that grows to about six to seven feet. They grow quite quickly, up to ten inches a year, so they are best suited to larger spaces. Areca palms also need bright, indirect sunlight and warm, humid air. Ideal temperatures for the areca palm are 65 to 70 degrees at night and 75 to 85 degrees during the day. They filter xylene and formaldehyde well and are useful in carpeted areas and near floors that have been newly varnished.
3. *Lady palm*. These palms have large, thick, shiny leaves. They are slow-growing and do well in bright, indirect sunlight. The top of the soil should be allowed to dry a bit between waterings (the exception is lady palms from Thailand, which need to be kept moist). Lady palms require a lot of space, as many types can grow to more than eight feet tall and wide.

Boston Fern

A fixture on the front porch and parlor rooms of Victorian homes, the Boston fern is a plant that works well in hanging baskets. Originating in tropical and subtropical regions of the world, it requires medium to bright indirect light, relatively cool temperatures, and lots of humidity. Although it needs to be watered regularly so that the soil stays moist, in the fall and winter months the soil can be allowed to dry somewhat between waterings. Boston ferns often require daily misting, so they are only for people who won't mind spending a few minutes each day with a spray bottle. They grow to about two feet in height.

Chinese Evergreen

If you don't have a green thumb, consider the Chinese evergreen, one of the most durable houseplants. They are easy to grow and tolerate low light and the dry air that's typical in many homes and offices. Chinese evergreens can grow up to three feet tall and three feet wide. They shouldn't be put into direct sunlight and the soil should be kept moist.

English Ivy

There are many varieties of this popular ivy. They filter out benzene, formaldehyde, and xylene, which makes them suitable near printers, computers, fax machines, plastic furniture, and new carpets and paint. You can place them in hanging baskets or on a high bookcase and allow them to grow down and around the shelves. Ivies usually continue to grow, so if they become too long, just prune them back. Smaller-leaved ivies tend to be slower growing. Ivy tends to grow well in areas that have plenty of bright, indirect light, although it can also grow in artificial light. They need to be thoroughly watered in pots that allow for good drainage.

Ficus

Ficus is a popular group of plants that reduce trichloroethylene, a chemical found in adhesives, paint removers, typewriter correction fluids, and spot removers. They are best suited to areas that receive direct sunlight for at least part of the day. The top of the soil should be allowed to dry slightly between waterings. The following three are among the most popular.

1. *Rubber plant.* A common houseplant with large, oval, dark green leaves.

2. *Weeping fig.* A popular house and office plant because it tolerates low humidity well. It can grow to about six to eight feet.
3. *Ficus alii.* This plant doesn't require quite as much water as other types of ficus. It has long, slender leaves.

Golden Pothos

Also called devil's ivy, golden pothos is an easy-to-grow plant with bright green leaves that will thrive in lower light conditions. It should be watered once a week. The golden pothos is a vine. You can trim its vines, root them, and then pot them in soil.

Peace Lily

The peace lily is one of the few green plants that grows in low light conditions and blooms periodically throughout the year. These sturdy plants are ideal for the office, where they can grow to up to four feet in height. Peace lilies filter many chemicals, including trichloroethylene, benzene, and formaldehyde. The dark green leaves have a graceful oval shape with pointy ends, and the flowers are a delicate white. The soil should be moist but allowed to dry somewhat between waterings; if it becomes too dry, the leaves will turn yellow along the edges. The plant also should not be over-watered. Although the peace lily can tolerate low light, the ideal conditions for it are bright, indirect light (it will burn in direct light).

Philodendron

There is a variety of philodendron, but the most common types have attractive, glossy, heart-shaped leaves. They grow best in medium, indirect sunlight, but can survive in lower light conditions. Direct sunlight, on the other hand, will burn the leaves.

Philodendron like humidity and should be misted regularly for optimal growth, but they will also tolerate the drier air found in most homes without misting. The soil should be kept moist but not soggy.

Spider Plant

The spider plant is one of the most common houseplants. It grows quickly to about two feet wide and three feet long, with miniature off-shoots that can be cut off and potted once they have roots, so you can easily fill your home with plants starting with just one. Spider plants need medium-to-bright indirect sunlight, so they should be placed near a window in a hanging basket. Move them away from the window in the winter so they don't become too cold. They should be allowed to dry slightly between waterings. Spider plants filter benzene and formaldehyde. They also filter carbon dioxide, which is why they are well suited to living rooms with fireplaces and kitchens with gas stoves.

Caution: If you have infants or pets, such as cats, make sure that the plants you have around your home are nontoxic to them. Peace lilies, philodendrons, golden pothos, and Chinese evergreens are toxic when ingested. Safer options are spider plants, lady palms, bamboo palms, and Boston ferns.

Keep a Food Journal

In 1993, the National Weight Control Registry began tracking the progress of more than three thousand people who maintained a weight loss of thirty pounds or more for at least a year. Participants report that one of their most important lessons was understanding that the key to achieving long-term success was finding a personalized program that fit them. Another important aspect was keeping a food journal. People who consistently keep track of what they eat stay with their programs for the long haul.

"Before I kept a journal, I'd think back to what I ate that day and just count the meals, and overlook all the snacking I did," confessed an office manager. "The first time I kept a three-day diet journal, I was shocked to see how much—and how poorly—I ate! Staff members are always bringing goodies to the office. A bite here, a bite there—it adds up. Keeping this journal was a real eye-opener."

This manager was right. It's easy to lose track of what you're eating when you're running from one obligation to the next. As cartoonist Bob Thaves said, "Inside me there's a thin person struggling to get out, but I can usually sedate him with four or five cupcakes." That's why it's so important to keep a food journal. Yes, it takes time, but it's an investment that will pay off for years to come because you will become more aware of those cupcakes and other snacks you may be using to comfort, sedate, and "treat" yourself.

A journal isn't just for recording food. It is an important tool that can guide you through this wonderful change in your life and help you with the psychological aspect of change. Gail Sheehy's *Pathfinders* was a land-mark book on how both men and women make and go through change in their lives. Sheehy describes two important steps.

1. *Develop an image of the future as you want it to be.* In the visualization section of your journal, write down anything that will help you develop your personal image of your health in the future.
2. *Develop a plan to reach your goal.* You have already made huge changes in your life. In the goals/plans section of your journal, write down your goals, no matter how large or small they may seem, and other plans for the future.

Every day, you'll come face to face with foods and situations that can make you forget why you are doing this. Taking a few minutes to affirm your goals and visualize your success will help guide you through the difficult days and keep them from throwing you off track. Following is a sample journal to give you ideas for what to include in yours.

Sample Journal

Date: May 28

Meals and Snacks

Breakfast	Had a blueberry smoothie on my way to work.
Lunch	Met Nancy for lunch. Ordered grilled organic chicken over a spinach salad with onions, squash, beets, and tomatoes. Cauliflower soup.
Snack(s)	Green tea, almonds, and apple slices.
Dinner	Thai curry with beans and veggies over brown rice with toasted flaxseeds.
Other Foods	Water and Other Beverages: _8_ glasses
	Super foods: Purple _1_ Orange _5_ White _2_ Cruciferous _2_ Omega yes Colon-cleansing _2_
	Flax: _2_ tablespoons Cleansing Lemon Tea: yes

Visualization

I am strong and determined.

Goals/Plans

To lose thirty pounds in six months. Increase my walk to sixty minutes.

Exercise

Thirty-minute walk with Nancy after lunch, thirty-minute exercise tape with ball and weights at 6 p.m.

Notes

Difficult client after lunch, cranky and stressed rest of the day. Energy crashed at 4 p.m.

Here are some tips for your journal.

- In the meals and snacks section, record any reason you ate besides hunger. You may also wish to note who you were with during the meal.
- For exercise, don't leave anything out. If you took the stairs, went for a brisk walk, hit the gym, record it. It all adds up!
- In the notes section, record any thoughts, challenges, emotions, events, or unusual circumstances. Were you traveling? Did you deal with a crisis at work or at home? Did you have a headache?

Your Journal

Date: May 28

Meals and Snacks

Breakfast

Lunch

Snack(s)

Dinner

Other Foods   Water and Other Beverages: ___ glasses
                        Super foods: Purple ___ Orange ___ White ___
                          Cruciferous ___ Omega ___ Colon-cleansing ___
                        Flax: ___ Cleansing Lemon Tea: ___

Visualization

Goals and Plans

Exercise

Notes

Cultivate a Supportive Circle

"I've had a horrible day," my client Janelle complained, plopping into the chair across from my desk. "My manager humiliated me in front of the project team today. He criticized me—in front of everyone—and said I had mishandled a sensitive negotiation. Then, this rude bank teller made me show two IDs to cash a check and I've been a customer at that bank for six years. I'm so steamed. I went home and worked my way through a pint of Ben and Jerry's."

Have you had days like that? We all have. That's when it's especially important to talk with someone who understands you. You may not want to broadcast it to the world, but it helps to get in touch with even just one person who knows what you're going through and will hold you accountable. That's why you can log on to www.iodiet.com at any time of the day to reach out to others who know exactly how you feel. There you will find an active forum, chats, and additional resources such as recipes and an online journal. You can also hear from people who have already turned their lives around by following the concrete steps in this program. Someone who has already made the journey can offer support to help you with yours.

12

Supplements

I went to a general store, but they wouldn't let me buy anything specific.
—COMEDIAN STEVEN WRIGHT

Although the only supplements that are recommended on the Inside Out Diet are a multivitamin and omega fatty acids, some people may wish to incorporate additional supplements into their daily routine. Some of the ones I'll discuss are not marketed as weight-loss supplements. Instead, they are aimed at keeping your body and mind in good working order, which allows your metabolism to become healthier and able to burn fat efficiently. These supplements are designed to support your liver, provide important nutrients, keep blood sugar levels steady, increase energy, balance hormones, decrease inflammation, and help manage stress.

Then there are the supplements meant strictly for weight loss. These include the fat-burners, appetite-suppressors, and metabolism-boosters. Although these supplements are popular and appealing, evidence shows that some are safer and more effective than others.

I certainly don't want you to take all of these supplements because they won't all be necessary or suitable for you. And some I suggest you avoid due to safety concerns. Besides, you are more likely to stick with a regular supplement routine if you take a few well-chosen supplements rather

than many. Use this list to learn what is available, and for addit...
ance in creating an individualized plan, consult a health practition...

Milk Thistle

Milk thistle has been used for liver and gallbladder disorders for more than two thousand years. A compound called silymarin in the seeds of the herb has been found to protect the liver from harmful substances and chemicals. Research shows that silymarin reduces fat accumulation in the liver, enhances detoxification, increases the synthesis of glutathione, and enhances the repair and regeneration of damaged liver cells. Milk thistle is also known as *Silybum marianum*, St. Mary's thistle, and Our Lady's Thistle. Look for extracts that have been standardized to 70 to 80 percent silymarin. Capsule or liquid extracts are better than tea because silymarin doesn't dissolve well in water. People with allergies to daisies, artichokes, kiwi, or plants in the aster family may have allergic reactions to milk thistle.

Side effects of milk thistle can include indigestion, headache, and itching. Milk thistle should be used with caution by people taking tranquilizers and antipsychotics. It shouldn't be used by people taking the herb yohimbe, or the blood pressure medication Regitine, as this herb counteracts the effects of both drugs. In theory, milk thistle may lower blood sugar levels, so people with hypoglycemia or diabetes should consult their doctor. Only the seed extract should be used, because the above-ground parts of the plant may have estrogenlike properties.

Alpha Lipoic Acid

Also called thioctic acid or lipoic acid, alpha lipoic acid is one of the few antioxidants that are soluble in both fat and water. Discovered in 1951, alpha lipoic acid is produced naturally in small amounts in the body. It helps cells generate energy and helps other antioxidants such as vitamins C and E work better. It has also been found to increase the production of glutathione, which aids in detoxification. Alpha lipoic acid is thought to enhance glucose metabolism and prevent or reverse the damage caused

e evidence supports this, but large, well-designed
use as a general antioxidant, a dosage of 20 to 50
mended.

riglycerides

Mediu... cerides (MCTs), also called fractionated coconut oil, belong to a special class of fatty acids. They are derived from coconut and palm-kernel oils. MCTs have become a popular weight-loss supplement because some studies have found that they can increase metabolism, resulting in increased fat-burning and weight loss. However, very large amounts must be taken. MCTs provide an immediate source of energy, which is why athletes take them to increase endurance. But again, great quantities must be consumed. I don't recommend this supplement because once ingested, MCTs are brought very quickly to the liver, which can put stress on the liver. Preliminary reports suggest that MCTs may raise cholesterol and triglycerides. People with liver disease, diabetes, and medium-chain acyl-coenzyme A dehydrogenase deficiency in particular should avoid MCTs.

Gymnema Sylvestre

Gymnema sylvestre is an ayurvedic herb that contains a sugarlike compound called gymnemic acid that is similar in chemical structure to glucose but has an opposite effect. Instead of raising blood sugar, gymnemic acid appears to bind to receptors in the intestines and decrease the uptake of glucose into the blood. A promising aspect of gymnema is that a preliminary study found it may be able to regenerate beta cells in the pancreas. It has been found to improve cholesterol and triglyceride levels.

Gymnema also contains a peptide called gurmarin that is believed to block the taste for sugar when the liquid extract is placed on the tongue. A typical dose starts at 50 mg to 150 mg three times a day. *Note*: Because it affects blood sugar levels, people taking diabetes medication should take gymnema under the supervision of a health practitioner because it could have an additive effect and cause a dangerous hypoglycemic reaction. Gymnema should not be used in place of insulin.

Chromium

Chromium is a trace mineral needed for normal protein, carbohydrate, and fat metabolism. One of chromium's main functions is to help insulin move glucose out of blood and into cells. Chromium deficiency is associated with hyperglycemia, hyperinsulinemia, and hypertriglyceridemia. It may aid weight loss in people who are glucose intolerant or insulin resistant by improving blood sugar and insulin, and it is believed to affect body composition by building lean muscle mass and burning fat. Although promising, three small randomized controlled trials examined the role of chromium for weight loss and did not find any difference between chromium and a placebo. Larger studies are needed.

Chromium picolinate, one of the most popular forms, has been linked with DNA damage in animal studies, which is why I prefer niacin-bound chromium, a form that has been shown to be well-absorbed and effective without the same toxicity concerns. In one study, it resulted in a significant loss of fat and sparing of muscle compared to a control group. People with diabetes or metabolic syndrome should get their doctor's approval before taking chromium. A typical amount used in weight-loss supplements is 200 micrograms.

Bitter Melon

Bitter melon (*Momordica charantia*) is a tropical fruit grown in South Asia, Southeast Asia, China, and the Caribbean. The fruit gets its name because it is one of the most bitter-tasting fruit. It looks like a very large, light-green bumpy cucumber. Compounds in bitter melon may work in a similar way to insulin. It has been used therapeutically to improve blood sugar regulation in people with type 2 diabetes. It should not be combined with diabetes medication except under supervision. There have been reports, however, that bitter melon may increase liver enzymes. Until we know more about the effects of bitter melon, I suggest holding off on using this fruit therapeutically.

Hoodia Gordonii

Hoodia gordonii is classified as a succulent, a cactuslike plant that can be found in Africa. The San Bushmen of the Kalahari desert, who live off the land, have been eating hoodia for a very long time, using it to ward off hunger and thirst during nomadic hunting trips. A study published in the September 2004 issue of *Brain Research* found that p57, believed to be the active compound in Hoodia, injected into the appetite center of rats' brains resulted in altered levels of adenosine triphosphate, an energy molecule that may affect hunger.

There is still very little published research on hoodia, however, and no long-term studies on its safety. Jasjit S. Bindra, Ph.D., a former researcher for hoodia at the pharmaceutical company Pfizer, stated in a letter to the *New York Times* that although hoodia did appear to suppress appetite, there were indications of unwanted effects on the liver caused by components other than the active ingredient that could not easily be removed through processing. It should be used with caution by people with diabetes because it may affect blood sugar levels. Hoodia may also interact with medications. The typical intake of hoodia is anywhere from 500 mg to 1,200 mg, taken with water one hour before meals. Hoodia is slow-growing, requiring four to five years to mature, so the demand for this plant is far ahead of the supply. This makes the quality and purity of hoodia supplements a concern.

Caralluma Fimbriata

Also believed to suppress appetite, *Caralluma fimbriata* is a succulent that grows wild in southern India and has been cooked like a vegetable, made into pickles and chutneys, and eaten raw for centuries by people in rural areas. Like hoodia, caralluma is believed to suppress appetite by affecting key brain centers. Caralluma contains pregnane glycosides, which researchers have postulated might prevent the formation of fat by blocking an enzyme called citrate lyase, which forces the body to burn stored fat. There is very little published research on this supplement. Caralluma may influence blood sugar levels, so it should be used with caution by people with diabetes.

Conjugated Linoleic Acid

Conjugated linoleic acid (CLA) is a family of trans-fatty acids that has been found to decrease fat deposition while preserving lean muscle. It is thought to inhibit lipoprotein lipase, an enzyme made by fat cells that's responsible for the uptake of fat by the cell. In two randomized controlled trials using 2 to 7 grams per day of CLA, however, there was no change in body mass index, but over 60 percent of subjects experienced mild to moderate digestive symptoms. More concerning is recent research indicating that the use of CLA in people with diabetes may lead to a worsening of blood sugar control. There are also concerns that it may worsen insulin sensitivity and increase the risk of heart disease in people who are overweight.

Hydroxycitric Acid

Hydroxycitric acid (HCA) is derived from *Garcinia cambogia*, a sour-tasting fruit native to India that is added to meals to make them more filling. Animal studies show that HCA reduces appetite and decreases calories stored as fat, although human studies don't always support these findings. HCA has been found to inhibit the enzyme citrate lyase and promote fat loss, without stimulating the central nervous system the way other popular weight-loss supplements do. It has also been found to improve glucose metabolism, has leptinlike activity, and increases serotonin release in animal studies. HCA appears to be well tolerated, with no known side effects or complications. A typical dose is 750 to 1,000 mg per day.

Bitter Orange

Also called *Citrus aurantium*, bitter orange is a fruit-derived extract. A compound in bitter orange called synephrine is chemically similar to ephedrine and believed to be responsible for the metabolism-boosting effect of the herb. However, bitter orange has been found to raise blood pressure and heart rate. Although most studies have involved intravenous administration, a placebo-controlled study at the University of California at San Francisco in which fifteen young, healthy subjects received either a 900 mg bitter-orange supplement, standardized to 6 percent synephrine, or a placebo found that blood pressure and heart rate were elevated for up to five hours after a single dose. Although the dose used was larger than the more typical 200 to 400 mg range, people should consult a health care provider before taking bitter orange, especially if they have heart disease, hypertension, or diabetes, or are taking any medication (bitter orange may cause interactions similar to grapefruit). Some supplements also contain green tea or other substances containing caffeine, which may augment the side effects.

Guarana

A plant originally from Brazil, guarana seeds have double the caffeine content of coffee beans. The caffeine in guarana is thought to be responsible for its ability to enhance fat metabolism. It also stimulates the central nervous system and heart, so guarana can cause anxiety and rapid heart rate in large amounts. People with high blood pressure and heart problems should avoid guarana. The FDA has recorded "adverse events" from the combination of bitter orange and caffeine, so avoid taking guarana with bitter orange. Guarana is a common ingredient in energy drinks and is also found in liquid and capsule forms, but keep in mind that it counts toward your daily caffeine intake, so find out how much caffeine is in each serving.

Yerba Mate

Yerba mate, a South American plant, has been found to reduce cholesterol and triglycerides in animal studies. In a study involving forty-seven people taking yerba mate and the herbs guarana and damiana for forty-five days, researchers reported that the group taking yerba mate felt satiated faster, showed an average weight loss of eleven pounds (compared to under one pound in the placebo group), and did not regain the weight during maintenance.

Yerba mate is rich in antioxidants and has also been found to inhibit the formation of advanced glycosylation end products, toxic substances that are produced when there are ongoing, high levels of sugars in the body.

Yerba mate contains caffeine, however, and may cause side effects such as increased blood pressure, heart rate, anxiety, and insomnia. More concerning is research linking yerba mate to esophageal cancer. Some of the risk appears to be reduced by drinking the tea in moderation and at a warm, not hot, temperature.

Chitosan

Chitosan is derived from chitin, found in the shells of crustaceans such as crabs and crayfish. It is believed to block the absorption of dietary fat from the intestines by binding with fat molecules, but studies have not confirmed this. A meta-analysis of fourteen trials involving 1,071 participants found little effect, especially when the analysis was limited to high-quality studies. The researchers concluded that "the effect of chitosan is minimal and unlikely to be of clinical significance." Another study found that with chitosan alone, it would take more than seven months to lose one pound of body fat.

Pyruvate

Pyruvate is a supplement popular with athletes and bodybuilders. It contains the compound pyruvic acid, which is important in energy metabolism. There is some evidence that pyruvate may help with weight loss and improve body composition. A six-week study using 6 grams of pyruvate per day was associated with weight loss, significant decreases in body fat, and increases in muscle mass compared with a placebo. A typical dose of pyruvate is 30 grams per day. A combination product called DHAP containing pyruvate and its precursor dihydroxyacetone can also be found. Side effects can include indigestion and diarrhea.

Senna

Commercial senna products are approved by the FDA for the treatment of occasional constipation. Senna contains chemicals such as anthraquinones, which work by impairing cells that line the colon. Long term use of senna products could lead to adverse effects commonly associated with laxatives, such as electrolyte imbalances. People taking digoxin or medications that deplete potassium such as thiazide or loop diuretics should avoid senna.

Cascara Sagrada

Another herb that is used as a laxative, cascara sagrada contains compounds called anthracene glycosides, which have been associated with chronic hepatitis. Reports have associated cascara sagrada with the development of cholestatic hepatitis.

Usnic Acid

Supplements containing usnic acid, derived from the lichen usnea, have been marketed for weight loss. Usnic acid supplements have been associated with liver toxicity, however. In one case report, a patient developed liver failure requiring emergency liver transplantation within three months of taking an usnic acid supplement. In another report, a patient developed liver necrosis, and no other cause of the liver damage besides usnic acid could be found.

5-HTP

The body uses 5-HTP to produce the neurotransmitter serotonin, so 5-HTP in supplement form is thought to boost the body's serotonin levels. The supplement is made from the seeds of an African plant called *Griffonia simplicifolia*. Although 5-HTP supplements are often used for depression, they have also been promoted for weight loss. Part of the rationale was that the weight-loss drug "fen-phen" raised serotonin levels, so other substances that boosted serotonin might also be helpful for weight loss. Studies have been promising. 5-HTP has been found to increase satiety, lower calorie intake (even though people made no effort to eat less), and reduce carbohydrate intake. 5-HTP should not be combined with drugs that raise serotonin levels, such as SSRI antidepressants, other antidepressants, migraine drugs in the triptan family, or the pain medication tramadol, except under medical supervision.

Enteric-Coated Peppermint Oil

Studies conducted over the last twenty years support the use of enteric-coated peppermint oil for irritable bowel syndrome symptoms; it's also been used to inhibit the growth of over twenty-two bacterial strains. It's particularly useful for bacterial overgrowth in the small intestine.

The words "enteric-coated" mean the capsules bypass your stomach and are only released once they reach your intestines, where they're needed, which also prevents heartburn, reflux, and other side effects. The typical dose used in research studies is 90 mg peppermint oil, often combined with 50 mg caraway in an enteric-coated capsule. It should be taken between meals.

Liquid Grapefruit Seed Extract

Grapefruit seed extract was first used by farmers to inhibit mold growth on their equipment. It became popular in the 1980s for its antifungal properties, but it also has general antimicrobial properties and is active against bacteria, fungi, and yeast, including *Candida albicans*, *Salmonella typhi*, *E. coli*, and *Giardia lamblia*. Not to be confused with grapeseed extract, grapefruit seed extract is derived from the seeds and pulp of grapefruit. It's also called citrus seed extract. The most popular form is liquid. A typical dose is two to three drops twice daily, between meals, in a glass of water. It should taste bitter. If it's too bitter to stomach, you've probably added too much, which over time can irritate or even damage the intestinal lining. Don't take grapefruit seed extract if you have citrus allergies. It may interact with medications, so the same precautions should be taken as with grapefruit juice.

Caprylic Acid

Caprylic acid is a natural eight-carbon fatty acid that's found in human and animal breast milk, possibly to protect infants from infection. The commercial preparation is derived from coconut and palm oil. It's a relatively clear liquid, which you can buy in bottles from a health food store. Caprylic acid has antimicrobial properties and is particularly active against *Candida albicans*. Undecylenate acid is another type of fatty acid that is used for this purpose. Typical doses are up to 3,500 mg caprylic acid a day and up to 1,000 mg undecylenate acid a day.

Oregano Oil

Oregano oil is an essential oil that has been distilled from oregano leaves. It contains the compound carvacrol, which has been found to be active against pathogenic intestinal microbes. Look for it in capsule form; it should not be taken as a liquid. It should be taken between meals with water. Do not take oregano oil if you are allergic to mint.

Digestive Enzymes

Enzyme supplements may be used to enhance digestion. They are especially useful in some cases of bloating and indigestion between meals. Pancreatic enzymes derived from animal sources are considered superior to vegetable-derived enzymes, because they are more similar to our own. It's important, however, to choose a quality source because it's animal derived. A typical dose is one to two capsules taken five to ten minutes before meals. They should not be chewed.

Cellulose

People with small-intestine bacterial overgrowth or intestinal permeability sometimes can't tolerate psyllium or even flaxseeds, even though they have a higher percentage of insoluble fiber. That's because some of the soluble fiber gets fermented by the unfriendly bacteria and worsens bloating. If bloating after taking fiber is a concern, a good choice would be cellulose. It promotes bowel movements and may help to heal intestinal permeability. Mix it as directed with water and drink.

Greens Powder

Chlorophyll, which is responsible for the green pigment in greens powder, is a potent detoxifier. Although gaining popularity in North America, greens powder is one of the most popular supplements in Japan, where it's ranked higher than vitamin C. An estimated five million people there take greens powder every day.

Although the powder has a dark green color, the taste is actually quite mild. It can be mixed into a small amount of water or into smoothies. The dark pigment of blueberries and blackberries usually can mask some of the green color. Greens powder is also available in tablet form and can be found at health food stores and some supermarkets. A typical daily dose during detoxification is 2 grams of greens powder. You can select one type of greens or use a combination of several. The most cost-effective approach is to take the powder (2 grams is about ½ to 1 teaspoon). Some people find capsules or tablets more convenient, although it's usually more costly and requires two to eight tablets to get 2 grams. When taking greens powder for the first time, start slowly and work up. Following are the different varieties of greens powder.

Chlorella: A First-Class Detoxifier

Chlorella, a freshwater single-celled algae, contains amino acids, vitamins, and minerals including beta-carotene and vitamin B12, fiber, a significant amount of chlorophyll, and chlorella growth factor, a concentrated source of DNA and RNA.

Chlorella helps protect the body against PCBs and toxins released from fat cells during weight loss. In Japan, chlorella is recommended to detoxify against PCBs. Following are some of chlorella's benefits.

- Detoxifies PCBs, bisphenol A, heavy metals such as mercury, and pesticides
- Absorbs toxins in the gut and ensures that they're excreted
- Improves friendly bacteria levels in the colon
- Reduces gas, bloating, and chronic constipation

Chlorella is also believed to prevent heart disease and cancer. Studies have found that it can reduce inflammation and lower blood pressure and cholesterol.

Note: The outer cell wall of chlorella is composed mainly of cellulose, which the human digestive tract can't effectively break down. When shopping for chlorella, look for "cracked cell" or "broken cell wall," which means the cell wall has been pulverized for better absorption of the chlorella. Some chlorella supplements contain vitamin K, which can reduce the effectiveness of the drug warfarin.

Blue-Green Algae

Blue-green algae, also known as Aphanizomenon flos-aquae, is a type of algae harvested from Upper Klamath Lake in southern Oregon and then freeze-dried and sold in powder, pill, and capsule forms. There have been concerns about blue-green algae products being contaminated with toxins called microcrystins that are harmful to the liver. The source of microcystins is another algae called Microcystis aeruginosa, which also grows in Upper Klamath Lake. One study looked at twelve supplements purchased over the Internet and found that all of them were contaminated. In the fall of 1996, the Oregon Health Division learned about the M. aeruginosa in Upper Klamath Lake and issued an advisory against water contact. It also established a safety limit for microcystins in blue-green algae products and tested eighty-seven products, of which 72 percent of the samples had a microcystin content that exceeded the safety limit.

Part IV

Recipes

All recipes and accompanying descriptive notes were created by celebrity chef Sabra Ricci unless otherwise indicated.

Breakfasts

Soups

Entrées

Snacks, Sauces, Dressings, and Beverages

Desserts

13

Recipes

Breakfasts

Asparagus Frittata   (Servings: 1)

A frittata is an Italian version of an omelet. Instead of being folded like an omelet, frittatas are usually open-faced or unfolded. This recipe captures the delicate flavor of asparagus. When buying asparagus, look for firm, bright green stalks with tightly closed tips. Don't wash asparagus before storing it. Just trim the ends of fresh asparagus and store them upright in the refrigerator in a container with about one inch of water at the bottom. Peel the ends of thicker stalks before cooking.

2 egg whites
olive oil spray
1 garlic clove, minced
¾ cup asparagus, cut on an angle into
  1-inch pieces, lightly steamed
⅛ cup sliced mushrooms

⅛ cup diced red pepper
2 tablespoons finely diced
  red onion
½ tablespoon minced basil
salt and pepper to taste
whole basil leaves (garnish)

Whisk the egg whites in a mixing bowl and set aside.

Spray a small skillet with olive oil. Add the garlic, asparagus, mushrooms, red pepper, onion, and basil. Sauté gently over medium heat until soft, about 5 minutes.

Gradually pour the egg whites over the sautéed vegetables. Lower the heat to medium and cook until the eggs are set and the underside is browned. Season with salt and pepper.

Gently transfer the frittata to a plate, turning it over so that the browned side is on top. Garnish with whole basil leaves. Serve hot.

Variation: Spray muffin tins lightly with olive oil and bake individual frittatas to eat on the run. You can also try substituting other vegetables for the asparagus.

Serving Ideas: Serve with a cup of green tea and Fruit Salad with Orange Mint Dressing (see the following recipe).

> Per Serving: 81 calories; trace fat; 10 g protein; 11 g carbohydrate; 4 g dietary fiber; 0 mg cholesterol; 114 mg sodium

Fruit Salad with Orange Mint Dressing   (Servings: 1)

Fresh fruit salad is a refreshing accompaniment to any dish. The colors of the fruits in this recipe are appealing to the eye, just as the blend of flavors is appealing to the palate.

When shopping for kiwi, determine the ripeness of the fruit by cupping one in your hand and gently squeezing. There should be a slight give to the pressure. If it feels mushy, it's overripe, and hardness indicates it is unripe. The pale green of the honeydew is a nice contrast, and the bright red and deep blue of the berries add the final touch, with a sweetness that bursts on the tongue. The citrus and mint in the dressing complete this wholesome treat.

1 kiwi, peeled and cut in wedges	¼ teaspoon finely grated lemon peel, preferably Meyer
¼ cup cubed honeydew	½ teaspoon fresh lemon juice, preferably Meyer
¼ cup sliced strawberries	
¼ cup blueberries	1 tablespoon fresh orange juice
½ tablespoon fresh mint	¼ teaspoon ground nutmeg

Combine the kiwi, honeydew, strawberries, and blueberries in a mixing bowl.

Place the remaining ingredients in a mini food processor; pulse until the mint is finely chopped.

Spoon the mixture over the fruit and stir gently until the fruit is coated.

> Per Serving: 104 calories; 1 g fat; 2 g protein; 25 g carbohydrate; 5 g dietary fiber; 0 mg cholesterol; 12 mg sodium

Pumpkin Pie Oatmeal   (Servings: 1)

This is a breakfast of many choices. You can use any of the allowed grains, including amaranth, barley, or oat groats. Try a single fruit, or combine your favorites. Add almond extract. It's all a matter of choice, as long as you stay within the guidelines.

1 cup water	½ cup canned pumpkin
pinch of salt	1 teaspoon pumpkin pie spice
½ cup old-fashioned oats	½ teaspoon vanilla extract

Place the water and salt in a small saucepan. Bring to a boil. Add the oats. Cook until most of the water is absorbed. Add the remaining ingredients. Mix well. Continue cooking until the oats are done.

Variation: Substitute applesauce and cinnamon for the pumpkin and pumpkin pie spice. Or substitute quinoa, millet, or buckwheat for the oatmeal. Add slivered almonds or chopped walnuts.

Variation: Using steel-cut oats instead of old-fashioned oats is another option. For a faster breakfast in the morning, start preparation the night before: boil the water and salt in a saucepan. Turn off the heat and add the steel-cut oats. Cover the saucepan and leave overnight. In the morning, add the remaining ingredients and cook until the oats are done.

Serving Ideas: Serve with a cup of green tea.

> Per Serving: 210 calories; 3 g fat; 8 g protein; 39 g carbohydrate; 8 g dietary fiber; 0 mg cholesterol; 16 mg sodium

Southwestern Egg Cups   (Servings: 6)

Specialty shops, health food stores, and the health food departments in major grocery chains carry many quality, tasty, low-calorie salsas. Try a smoky chipotle pepper salsa or one with fire-roasted tomatoes. Adding 1 to 2 teaspoons of ground flaxseeds would be a nice addition to any variation. Freeze extra egg cups individually for breakfast or lunch on the run. Leftover egg cups can be stored in the freezer for up to two weeks.

olive oil spray	½ cup finely chopped roasted pepper
24 egg whites	1 can green chilies, diced
1 medium onion, finely chopped	1 teaspoon oregano
1 can low-sodium black beans	sea salt and pepper to taste

Preheat the oven to 325°.

Rinse the beans well and drain.

Spray a 6-cup muffin tin with olive oil. Set aside.

Beat the egg whites until frothy. Set aside.

Spray a medium skillet with olive oil. Add the onions and sauté until translucent. Cool slightly.

Add the onions and all other ingredients to the egg whites. Mix well.

Fill the muffin cups to ¾ full. Bake for 12 minutes or until the egg whites are set.

Serving Ideas: Top with your favorite low-calorie salsa.

> Per Serving: 84 calories; trace fat; 15 g protein; 5 g carbohydrate; 1 g dietary fiber; 0 mg cholesterol; 245 mg sodium

Raspberry Almond Smoothie   (Servings: 1)

8 ounces almond milk, low-fat
⅔ ounce vanilla whey protein
  powder

½ cup raspberries
¼ teaspoon almond extract
¼ cup crushed ice

Combine all the ingredients in a blender. Blend until smooth.

Variation: Substitute any allowed fruit for the raspberries. Instead of the almond extract, try spices such as cinnamon, nutmeg, allspice, or a combination.

> Per Serving: 177 calories; 3.2 g fat; 17 g protein; 19.9 g carbohydrate; 4.2 g dietary fiber; 15 mg cholesterol; 148 mg sodium

Candied Sweet Potato   (Servings: 2)

Baking the sweet potato in a microwave may be faster, but there's nothing quite like the taste and smell of oven-roasted sweet potatoes. For a quick breakfast, prepare this recipe the night before in the oven and then reheat it in the microwave in the morning. It can also be transported easily for lunch.

olive oil spray
1 medium sweet potato, scrubbed
1 tablespoon toasted chopped pecans
1 teaspoon toasted ground flaxseeds

2 teaspoons almond butter
1 teaspoon stevia or other natural
  sweetener
cinnamon

Preheat the oven to 400°. Spray a small baking sheet with olive oil.

Trim off the ends of the sweet potato and place it on the baking sheet. Bake the sweet potato for 50 to 60 minutes or until soft.

Split the sweet potato in half lengthwise. With a fork, mash and fluff the insides of one half of the sweet potato. (Wrap and save one half in the refrigerator or freezer for another meal.)

Add the pecans, flaxseeds, almond butter, and stevia to the sweet potato. Sprinkle with cinnamon.

Time-saving Tip: Cook the sweet potato in the microwave for 5 to 8 minutes instead of baking it in the oven.

> Per Serving: 136 calories; 5 g fat; 3 g protein; 19 g carbohydrate; 3 g dietary fiber; 0 mg cholesterol; 10 mg sodium

Cherry Kefir Smoothie   (Servings: 1)

1 cup low-fat plain kefir
2/3 ounce plain or vanilla whey protein
  powder
1/2 cup frozen pitted sweet cherries

1 teaspoon stevia, or to taste
1/2 teaspoon cinnamon
1/4 cup crushed ice

Combine all the ingredients in a blender. Blend until smooth.

Variation: Try yogurt as a substitute for the kefir. Add extra ice, 1/4 cup water, or nut milk to thin the yogurt.

> Per Serving: 283 calories; 1 g fat; 28 g protein; 49 g carbohydrate; 5 g dietary fiber; 4 mg cholesterol; 190 mg sodium

Eggs Florentine   (Servings: 1)

This is a healthy variation on the classic eggs benedict, without the added fat and calories. When selecting the tomato, or any fruit or vegetable for that matter, one of the best guidelines for taste and flavor is how it smells. You want a tomato that smells like a tomato. If you can't recognize the tomato fragrance when you close your eyes and someone places a tomato under your nose, it's not going to taste like a tomato. So let your nose do the shopping.

1 beefsteak tomato, sliced into
  1-inch-thick slices
1 cup fresh spinach
1 teaspoon olive oil

1 teaspoon lemon juice
1 whole egg
salt and pepper to taste

Place 1 tomato slice on a plate. Salt to taste.

Sauté the spinach in olive oil and lemon juice in a skillet, about 5 minutes.

Poach the egg.

Place the spinach on top of the tomato slice. Transfer the egg to the top of the spinach pile. Add the salt and pepper. Garnish with the remaining tomato slices.

Serving Ideas: Serve with a 2-inch cantaloupe wedge, ½ cup raspberries, and 1 cup tea, herbal or black.

> Per Serving: 122 calories; 10 g fat; 7 g protein; 2 g carbohydrate; 1 g dietary fiber; 212 mg cholesterol; 94 mg sodium

Scrambled Egg Oatmeal   (Servings: 1)

1 egg	½ cup old-fashioned oatmeal
1 cup water	⅔ ounce plain protein powder
pinch of salt	

Beat the egg in a small bowl. Set aside.

Place the water in a small saucepan. Add a pinch of salt and bring it to a boil. Add the oatmeal and cook until the water is absorbed. Add the egg and protein powder and stir constantly until egg is cooked.

> Per Serving: 268 calories; 8 g fat; 20 g protein; 28 g carbohydrate; 6 g dietary fiber; 212 mg cholesterol; 79 mg sodium

Muesli Cereal   (Servings: 1)

(Recipe by Cathy Wong)

¾ cup almond milk, low-fat	1 tablespoon toasted ground flaxseeds
1 tablespoon vanilla whey protein powder	1 tablespoon sliced almonds
⅓ cup toasted oats	¼ cup blackberries

Mix the almond milk and whey protein powder in a bowl until smooth. Add the oats and soak overnight.

In the morning, top with the remaining ingredients and serve.

> Per Serving: 415 calories; 13.9 g fat; 19.7 g protein; 52.9 g carbohydrate; 10.7 g dietary fiber; 6 mg cholesterol; 100 mg sodium

Blueberry Flax Cereal   (Servings: 1)

(Recipe by Cathy Wong)

2 tablespoons flaxseeds
½ cup almond milk, low-fat
1 tablespoon vanilla whey protein
  powder

¾ cup blueberries
1 tablespoon sliced almonds

Toast the flaxseeds in an oven at 250° for 10 to 15 minutes. Remove from the oven and set aside. In a bowl, mix the almond milk with the protein powder until smooth. Add the blueberries. Top with the almonds. Add the flaxseeds and serve immediately.

Per Serving: 289 calories; 13.9 g fat; 12.7 g protein; 29.9 g carbohydrate; 8.9 g dietary fiber; 6 mg cholesterol; 83 mg sodium

Berry Smoothie   (Servings: 1)

(Recipe by Cathy Wong)

¾ cup frozen berries (e.g., raspberry,
  blueberry, blackberry)
½ cup low-fat vanilla yogurt

½ cup cold water
1 scoop vanilla whey protein
  powder

Combine all the ingredients in a blender. Blend until smooth. Pour into a glass and serve.

Per Serving: 212 calories; 1.1 g fat; 23.7 g protein; 26.8 g carbohydrate; 2.9 g dietary fiber; 19 mg cholesterol; 149 mg sodium

Two-Minute Omelet   (Servings: 1)

(Recipe by Cathy Wong)

2 egg whites
⅛ teaspoon turmeric
1 tablespoon low-fat coconut milk
½ cup frozen chopped spinach

1 slice cooked turkey bacon,
  chopped
½ cup finely diced red pepper
1 teaspoon chopped fresh basil

Mix the egg whites, turmeric, and low-fat coconut milk in a 1-cup ramekin or a small bowl. Add the remaining ingredients. Cover and microwave for 2 minutes.

Variation: You can try this with other vegetables, such as mushrooms, asparagus tips, spinach, and artichokes.

> Per Serving: 114 calories; 2.3 g fat; 14.4 g protein; 8.8 g carbohydrate; 3.8 g dietary fiber; 15 mg cholesterol; 372 mg sodium

Flaxseed Granola   (Servings: 22)

(Recipe by Cathy Wong)

4 cups old-fashioned rolled oats
1½ cups ground flaxseeds
1½ teaspoons ground cinnamon
1½ teaspoons ground ginger
5 tablespoons blackstrap molasses
⅓ cup almond or grapeseed oil

¼ cup water
½ cup unsweetened dry coconut
  flakes
¾ cup almonds
¾ cup chopped walnuts

Place the oven rack in the center position of the oven. Preheat the oven to 300°.

In a large mixing bowl, combine the oats, flaxseeds, cinnamon, and ginger.

In a separate small bowl, mix together the molasses, oil, and water. Pour this over the oat mixture and stir it until the oat mixture is fully coated.

Cover a large baking sheet with foil and spread the mixture evenly.

Bake the granola in the oven for about 45 minutes, stirring halfway through, until the mixture is dry and evenly cooked. Allow it to cool to room temperature.

In a large bowl, combine the oat mixture, coconut flakes, almonds, and walnuts. Pour the mixture into an airtight container and store at room temperature for up to one month.

> Per Serving: 281 calories; 15.1 g fat; 8.4 g protein; 27.7 g carbohydrate; 6.8 g dietary fiber; 0 mg cholesterol; 46 mg sodium

Soups

Black Bean and Pumpkin Soup with Chicken   (Servings: 4)

Black beans are also called turtle beans. They have a creamy flesh surrounded by a smooth, shiny black skin. The taste is slightly sweet. These beans are perfect for soups. Canned pumpkin was chosen for this soup for a consistent texture. Fresh pumpkin would work as well, but certain varieties have a higher water content and do not cook down easily to a thick puree.

It is best to use organic chicken whenever possible. The soup may be transported in a thermos to keep it hot, or bring it to work and reheat it in a microwave. Freeze the extra soup in individual containers for a later date.

1 small onion, chopped	1 tablespoon cumin
1 clove garlic, minced	2 teaspoons pumpkin pie spice
1 tablespoon olive oil	dash cayenne
1 can black beans	1 smoked chipotle pepper in adobo
1 can plain diced tomatoes	sauce
1 can pumpkin	1 small chicken breast, thinly sliced

Rinse the beans well and drain.

Sauté the onion and garlic in olive oil in a large saucepan over medium heat for 2 to 4 minutes. Add the remaining ingredients, except the chicken. Simmer covered for about 10 minutes.

While the soup is cooking, spray a skillet with olive oil and sauté the chicken until it is no longer pink, about 5 minutes. Set it aside and keep warm.

Pour the soup into a blender and blend until smooth. Return the soup to the saucepan and add the chicken. Reheat to the desired temperature.

Ladle the soup into serving bowls.

Serving Ideas: Serve with a side salad of spinach with extra-virgin olive oil and lemon.

> Per Serving: 297 calories; 5 g fat; 25 g protein; 38 g carbohydrate; 9 g dietary fiber; 34 mg cholesterol; 49 mg sodium

Barley-Lentil Soup with Swiss Chard   (Servings: 4)

Lentils are used as a substitute for meat throughout India, parts of Europe, and the Middle East. They are not eaten fresh, but are dried upon ripening, so they are a staple that can be stored in your pantry for up to a year. Barley has been used since the Stone Age in a variety of foods and beverages from spirits to bread. This is a hearty, satisfying dish. Serve it with Chopped Salad for a nice combination of textures—the warm, smooth and creamy soup, with the cool, crisp and crunchy salad.

½ can lentils
olive oil spray
½ cup chopped onion
½ cup chopped celery
2 cloves minced garlic
1 cup water
1½ tablespoons finely minced

fresh thyme
1 teaspoon ground cumin
1 cup cooked barley
1 can diced tomatoes
3 cups low-sodium vegetable broth
sea salt and pepper to taste
2 cups coarsely chopped Swiss chard

Rinse the lentils well and drain.

Spray a stockpot with olive oil. Add the onion, celery, and garlic and sauté for 2 to 3 minutes.

Add all the remaining ingredients, except the Swiss chard, and simmer for 7 to 8 minutes. Add the Swiss chard and simmer until the chard is cooked.

Serving Ideas: Serve with Chopped Salad (see the recipe on page 204). Extra soup can be frozen in individual servings for later.

Per Serving: 304 calories; 2 g fat; 22 g protein; 54 g carbohydrate; 18 g dietary fiber; 0 mg cholesterol; 454 mg sodium

Super Green Chicken Soup   (Servings: 4)

2 boneless, skinless chicken breasts
1 leek, white and light green parts, chopped
1 cup chopped celery
1 cup chopped cabbage
2 cups organic chicken broth
1 cup water

1 clove garlic, minced
1 bay leaf
1 tablespoon chopped fresh parsley
pepper to taste
1 cup kale
1 cup Swiss chard

Combine all the ingredients in a small stock pot except the kale and Swiss chard. Simmer until the chicken is done.

Remove the chicken and set it aside to cool. Add the kale and Swiss chard. Lower the heat and continue cooking.

Cube the chicken and return it to the pot. Simmer just until the chicken is reheated. Remove the bay leaf.

Extra servings can be frozen for later.

Per Serving: 190 calories; 2 g fat; 34 g protein; 9 g carbohydrate; 2 g dietary fiber; 68 mg cholesterol; 399 mg sodium

Watercress and Leek Soup   (Servings: 4)

4 leeks   2 cups low-sodium chicken broth
4 cups watercress   ½ cup plain yogurt (omit in step 1)

Wash the leeks thoroughly to remove any dirt from the stems. Remove the dark green stems and discard them. Finely chop the leeks.

In a small stockpot, combine the leeks, watercress, and chicken broth. Simmer until the vegetables are cooked.

Remove the pot from the heat and cool slightly. Blend the soup in a blender or with a handheld immersion blender until smooth.

Return the soup to the pot. Add the yogurt, if using. Simmer until the soup is reheated.

Extra portions can be frozen for later.

Variation: Those who need a nondairy alternative can try soy yogurt.

Per Serving: 102 calories; 1 g fat; 9 g protein; 15 g carbohydrate; 2 g dietary fiber; 4 mg cholesterol; 305 mg sodium

Brussels Sprouts Soup   (Servings: 4)

Brussels sprouts were first cultivated in Belgium more than five hundred years ago. They look like miniature cabbages, so it's no surprise that they are in the cabbage family. But unlike cabbage, Brussels sprouts are slightly bitter. They taste wonderful, as long as they're not overcooked.

1 small onion, diced   ½ teaspoon minced garlic
1 celery stalk, diced   1 teaspoon chopped fresh thyme
1 small carrot, diced   2 cups low-sodium organic chicken or
1 small red pepper, diced   vegetable stock
½ pound Brussels sprouts   salt and pepper to taste

Add all the ingredients in a medium pot and bring to a boil. Reduce the heat and simmer until the Brussels sprouts are tender, about 20 minutes.

Puree half the soup in a blender and return it to the soup pot.

Freeze any remaining soup for later.

Per Serving: 76 calories; trace fat; 8 g protein; 12 g carbohydrate; 5 g dietary fiber; 0 mg cholesterol; 288 mg sodium

Jerusalem Artichoke and Leek Soup   (Servings: 4)

¾ pound Jerusalem artichokes
2 leeks
4 cups low-sodium chicken
  broth

2 cups water
1 cup plain soymilk
1 teaspoon thyme
1 teaspoon pepper

Scrub the artichokes. Peels can be left on, but remove any tough ends or peel completely if desired.

Wash the leeks carefully to remove any dirt trapped between the layers of the stem. Use only the white and light green parts. Finely chop the leeks.

In a small stockpot combine artichokes, leeks, chicken broth, and 1 cup of the water. Cook until the artichokes are tender. Add the remaining water as necessary during cooking. Remove from the heat and cool slightly. Blend the soup until smooth in a blender or with a handheld immersion blender.

Return the soup to the pot. Add the soymilk, thyme, and pepper. Simmer until the soup thickens and the flavors are blended.

Freeze the remaining soup in individual servings for later.

Variation: Substitute rice milk for the soymilk. Add a bay leaf or your favorite seasoning.

> Per Serving: 110 calories; 1g fat; 10 g protein; 16 g carbohydrate; 2 g dietary fiber; 0 mg cholesterol; 361 mg sodium

Entrées

Chicken Stir-Fry over "Rice"   (Servings: 1)

Nearly everyone loves stir-fry over rice, but the carbohydrate content in rice can be too high for some people. The "rice" in this recipe creates the illusion of the complete stir-fry meal without all those carbs. The blending of the vegetables and chicken with traditional stir-fry seasonings is the perfect topping for the "rice." The shredding blade of the food processor will cut just the right-size pieces of cauliflower. By steaming them until just tender the texture will be similar to that of cooked rice.

1 teaspoon low-sodium soy sauce or tamari

3 tablespoons water

1 teaspoon sesame oil

1 tablespoon olive oil

1 teaspoon minced garlic

1 teaspoon minced fresh ginger

1 boneless, skinless chicken breast, thinly sliced

pinch arrowroot

½ small onion, cut into thin wedges

½ cup sliced mushrooms

6 asparagus spears, sliced on the diagonal into 1-inch pieces

8 snowpea pods, strings removed, sliced on the diagonal into 1-inch pieces

¼ head cauliflower, shredded, using a food processor shredding blade

Mix the soy sauce or tamari, water, and sesame oil in a small bowl and set aside.

Heat the olive oil in a wok, if available, or a frying pan. Add the garlic, ginger, and chicken and stir-fry for 3 to 4 minutes. Thicken the juices slightly by mixing in a pinch of arrowroot.

Add the onion, mushrooms, asparagus, pea pods, and the soy sauce mixture to the pan. Simmer for 2 to 4 minutes until the asparagus is bright green, tender, and crisp.

While the stir-fry is cooking, steam the cauliflower "rice" until it is tender. Do not overcook. Drain the "rice" and transfer it to a plate or a glass container. Top it with the stir-fry and serve it immediately, or pack it so you can reheat it later in a microwave. This is an easily transported lunch.

Serving Ideas: Serve with a cup of tea and a piece of fruit, such as kiwi, tangerine, or guava.

Per Serving: 467 calories; 18 g fat; 60 g protein; 16 g carbohydrate; 5 g dietary fiber; 137 mg cholesterol; 369 mg sodium

Black-Eyed Pea Stew (Servings: 1)

Black beans and collard greens are both good sources of vitamins A and C, with the beans adding protein and the collards supplying calcium and iron. They blend together well and are used in the cuisine of several cultures. Collards peak between January and April, but they can usually be found year round. Leaves should be green and crisp, with no yellowing or wilting evident.

1 can black-eyed peas
½ onion, medium dice
1 carrot, peeled, medium dice
1 ripe tomato, peeled, cored, and
  chopped
1 celery stalk, sliced
1 clove garlic, minced
1 teaspoon dried thyme

pinch red pepper flakes
1 bay leaf
1 cup low-salt chicken or vegetable
  stock
½ pound collard greens or more,
  · chopped
salt and pepper to taste
⅓ cup plain yogurt (omit in step 1)

Rinse and drain the black-eyed peas and place them in a medium-size heavy saucepan together with the onion, carrot, tomato, celery, garlic, thyme, red pepper flakes, and bay leaf.

Stir in the stock and place the pan over moderately high heat. Bring to a boil, uncovered, about 3 minutes. Lower the heat and allow it to simmer uncovered for 10 minutes.

Add the collard greens and season with salt and pepper. Cook, uncovered, for 5 minutes or longer. Discard the bay leaf. Before serving, top with the yogurt.

Variation: For those who need a nondairy alternative, try soy yogurt.

Serving Ideas: Serve with Arugula Salad (see the following recipe).

Per Serving: 411 calories; 3 g fat; 31 g protein; 70 g carbohydrate; 16 g dietary fiber; 5 mg cholesterol; 351 mg sodium

Arugula Salad   (Servings: 1)

Arugula, also known as rocket, has a slightly bitter, aromatic taste. It can be too pungent for some palates, but the baby greens in this recipe sweeten the taste. You can also use tangerines, clementines, and satsumas. Satsumas are virtually seedless, so they are the nicest segments for this salad.

1 cup arugula
1 cup baby greens
1 mandarin orange, segmented
10 pecan halves, chopped

2 teaspoons olive oil
½ to 1 teaspoon balsamic vinegar, to
  taste

Combine all the ingredients in a large mixing bowl. Toss well.

Per Serving: 216 calories; 19 g fat; 2 g protein; 13 g carbohydrate; 3 g dietary fiber; 0 mg cholesterol; 6 mg sodium

Grilled Chicken Breast   (Servings: 1)

The chicken in combination with Zucchini Medley and Roasted Vegetable Salsa has received accolades. The presentation is very nice and easy to arrange.

1 small boneless, skinless chicken
  breast
1 teaspoon finely minced fresh
  thyme

juice of ½ lemon
½ clove garlic, finely minced
1 tablespoon olive oil

Combine all the ingredients in a bowl and cover. Marinate for 2 hours. (This can be done ahead of time.)

Remove the chicken and drain the excess oil. Grill for 5 or 6 minutes on each side.

Serving Ideas: Serve on a bed of Zucchini Medley (see the following recipe) topped with Roasted Vegetable Salsa (see the recipe below).

Per Serving: 386 calories; 16 g fat; 55 g protein; 2 g carbohydrate; trace dietary fiber; 137 mg cholesterol; 154 mg sodium

Zucchini Medley   (Servings: 1)

Small, slender zucchini have thinner skins, so they will be more tender and less bitter.

olive oil spray
1 small zucchini, grated

1 small yellow squash, grated
1 small white onion, thinly sliced

Spray a skillet with olive oil. Add the vegetables and sauté until tender, about 7 minutes. Transfer to a plate and serve.

Per Serving: 94 calories; 1 g fat; 5 g protein; 20 g carbohydrate; 7 g dietary fiber; 0 mg cholesterol; 12 mg sodium

Roasted Vegetable Salsa   (Servings: 1)

This salsa can also be served with a variety of meat or vegetable dishes.

1 cup grape tomatoes, halved
1 small Maui onion, or other sweet
  white onion (e.g., Vidalia, Walla
  Walla, or Oso)

handful of basil leaves
½ cup red pepper, cut into thin strips
kosher salt to taste
1 tablespoon olive oil

Preheat the oven to 400°.

Combine all the ingredients in a bowl. Mix well.

Transfer to a baking dish and bake for 20 minutes.

> Per Serving: 217 calories; 14 g fat; 4 g protein; 22 g carbohydrate; 5 g dietary fiber; 0 mg cholesterol; 19 mg sodium

Chopped Salad   (Servings: 1)

1½ cups chopped romaine lettuce
½ cup peeled and chopped
  cucumber
¼ cup chopped tomato

¼ cup chopped red onion
1 teaspoon olive oil
juice of ½ lemon
sea salt and pepper to taste

Toss all the ingredients in a large salad bowl until well mixed. Transfer to a plate or a serving bowl.

> Per Serving: 84 calories; 5 g fat; 3 g protein; 9 g carbohydrate; 3 g dietary fiber; 0 mg cholesterol; 13 mg sodium

Sweet Potato with Curried Vegetables   (Servings: 1)

Sweet potatoes are a nice alternative to white potatoes, whether baked, boiled, or sautéed. They work equally well as an entrée or a side dish.

1 large sweet potato, peeled and
  chopped into 1-inch pieces
water
pinch of sea salt
½ cup chopped white onion
½ cup chopped red bell pepper
1 cup chopped zucchini

¼ cup low-sodium vegetable
  broth
¼ low-fat coconut milk
⅛ teaspoon green curry paste
1 teaspoon minced lemongrass
1 teaspoon minced ginger
sea salt and pepper to taste

Put the sweet potato, salt, and enough water to cover the potato into a saucepan. Boil on medium heat until tender, about 20 minutes.

Place all the remaining ingredients in a skillet and simmer until the vegetables are tender.

Drain the sweet potato and mash it with a small amount of sea salt and pepper. Transfer it to a plate and top with the vegetables.

Serving Ideas: Serve with sliced peaches and raspberries.

> Per Serving: 217 calories; 14 g fat; 4 g protein; 22 g carbohydrate; 5 g dietary fiber; 0 mg cholesterol; 19 mg sodium

Grilled Turkey Breast Cutlet   (Servings: 1)

The Grilled Turkey Breast Cutlet is the right amount of protein to be served with Mixed Baby Greens with Blood Oranges, Almonds, and Pomegranates, a rather exotic salad. Removing the tiny seeds of the pomegranate from the whole fruit can be a challenge, but now you can find the seeds in small containers at a variety of specialty shops, including Trader Joe's, during the fall season. Blood oranges have a sweet-tart taste like many regular oranges, but with their deep red flesh, they make a dramatic addition to dishes. They are best eaten fresh, although one variety, the Maltese, works well cooked in a sauce.

1 teaspoon lemon juice
1 teaspoon olive oil
½ small shallot, minced
1 teaspoon cranberry sauce

sea salt and freshly ground pepper to taste
3-ounce turkey breast cutlet

Combine the lemon juice, olive oil, shallot, cranberry sauce, salt, and pepper in small bowl and whisk together. Add the turkey breast cutlet to the bowl, cover, and marinate for 20 minutes.

Grill the cutlet until it is no longer pink inside, about 4 minutes on each side, basting with marinade. Do not overcook. Transfer it to a serving plate.

Serving Ideas: Serve with 4 spears steamed asparagus and Mixed Baby Greens with Blood Oranges, Almonds, and Pomegranates (see the following recipe).

Per Serving: 138 calories; 6 g fat; 18 g protein; 4 g carbohydrate; trace dietary fiber; 48 mg cholesterol; 172 mg sodium

Mixed Baby Greens with Blood Oranges, Almonds, and Pomegranates   (Servings: 1)

2 blood oranges (1 cut into segments and 1 cut in half for the dressing)
1 cup mixed baby greens
1 cup arugula
1 tablespoon toasted almonds, slivered

2 tablespoons pomegranate seeds
½ tablespoon unseasoned rice vinegar
1 tablespoon olive oil
salt and pepper to taste

Combine the blood orange segments, baby greens, arugula, almonds, and pomegranate seeds in a salad bowl and set aside.

To make the dressing, squeeze 1 tablespoon of blood orange juice from the remaining orange and whisk together with the remaining ingredients in a separate bowl. Pour the dressing over the salad and lightly toss to coat. Transfer the salad to a plate and serve.

> Per Serving: 178 calories; 18 g fat; 2 g protein; 3 g carbohydrate; 1 g dietary fiber; 0 mg cholesterol; 6 mg sodium

Brown Rice with Kale   (Servings: 1)

½ cup brown rice   1 cup coarsely chopped kale
1 cup water   1 teaspoon olive oil
pinch of sea salt   juice of ½ lemon

Place the rice, water, and salt in a saucepan. Bring to a boil, reduce the heat, cover, and simmer for about 50 minutes.

Sauté the kale in the olive oil and lemon juice until tender. Transfer the kale to a plate and place the rice on the kale.

Serving Ideas: Top this dish with 1 cup of Vegetarian Chili (see the following recipe).

> Per Serving: 421 calories; 8 g fat; 9 g protein; 80 g carbohydrate; 3 g dietary fiber; 0 mg cholesterol; 40 mg sodium

Vegetarian Chili   (Servings: 4)

1 can kidney beans   ½ teaspoon chili powder
1 can garbanzo beans   1 teaspoon cumin
1 small white onion, chopped   1 cup water
2 roma tomatoes, chopped   sea salt to taste

Rinse the beans well and drain.

Add all the ingredients to a saucepan. Simmer until the chili has cooked down to a thick consistency, about 25 minutes.

Freeze the remaining chili in individual servings for a later date.

Serving Ideas: Serve with Brown Rice with Kale (see the previous recipe).

> Per Serving: 361 calories; 4 g fat; 21 g protein; 64 g carbohydrate; 21 g dietary fiber; 0 mg cholesterol; 35 mg sodium

Grilled Beef Tenderloin Salad   (Servings: 1)

This dish has an Asian influence with the blending of all these flavors.

1 clove garlic, finely minced
juice of 1 lemon
1 teaspoon soy sauce
cracked black pepper to taste
3 ounces beef tenderloin
1 cup chopped romaine lettuce
½ cup shredded red cabbage

½ cup shredded napa cabbage
½ cup sunflower sprouts
¼ white onion, thinly sliced
⅛ avocado, cubed
¼ cup thinly sliced radishes
2 teaspoons olive oil
sea salt and pepper to taste

Combine the garlic, half the lemon juice, soy sauce, and pepper in a bowl and cover. Add the beef and marinate overnight.

Combine all the vegetables in a large mixing bowl and toss to mix well.

Combine the rest of the lemon juice, olive oil, salt, and pepper in a small bowl and set aside.

Grill the beef to the desired doneness. Remove from the grill and allow it to rest for 5 minutes. Slice on a diagonal in ½-inch slices.

Toss the salad with the dressing. Transfer it to a plate and top with the beef slices.

> Per Serving: 669 calories; 42 g fat; 30 g protein; 49 g carbohydrate; 16 g dietary fiber; 60 mg cholesterol; 261 mg sodium

Curried Chicken Salad in Lettuce Wrap   (Servings: 1)

A chicken salad sandwich or a tortilla wrap is a great lunch, whether it is a traditional chicken salad or this curried version. This lettuce wrap is a nice alternative to bread or a tortilla. Cranberries and pecans offer an unexpected taste and texture not usually found in chicken salads. The dark red berries are referred to as bounceberries, because ripe ones bounce right off the vine. Try eating them to put a bounce in your step.

3 ounces boneless, skinless chicken
  breast, precooked and cut in
  ½-inch cubes
¼ cup diced celery
1 tablespoon dried cranberries
10 pecan halves, toasted and
  chopped

1 tablespoon finely chopped red
  onion
1 tablespoon low-fat mayonnaise
½ teaspoon curry powder
¼ teaspoon sea salt
⅛ teaspoon pepper
3 to 4 butter lettuce leaves

Combine all the ingredients except the lettuce leaves in a large mixing bowl. Mix well to allow the flavors to combine.

Arrange the lettuce leaves on a cutting board, overlapping the edges to form a "wrap" for the chicken salad. Scoop the chicken salad onto the lettuce leaves about 2 to 3 inches from one edge. Fold the 2- to-3-inch lettuce flap over the chicken and tightly roll to form a wrap. Secure with toothpicks.

Serving Ideas: Serve with green and red pepper strips, sliced cucumbers, and a cup of herbal tea.

> Per Serving: 303 calories; 23 g fat; 22 g protein; 6 g carbohydrate; 3 g dietary fiber; 54 mg cholesterol; 164 mg sodium

Chicken Egg Fu Yung with Fried "Rice" (Servings: 1)

You are guaranteed no MSG when you indulge in this tasty and easy-to-prepare dish. It will be reminiscent of your favorite restaurant dish without the calories, fats, or carbs, and you don't even have to leave home. You can easily substitute other protein sources or vegetables, or turn leftovers into an interesting meal.

1 jumbo egg
1 teaspoon low-sodium soy sauce
olive oil spray
¼ teaspoon finely minced fresh
  ginger
2-ounce chicken breast, precooked,
  finely shredded
½ cup finely shredded Chinese
  cabbage
½ cup bean sprouts
⅛ cup finely sliced green onion

⅛ cup finely chopped mushrooms
⅛ cup finely chopped water
  chestnuts
1 teaspoon olive oil
4 green onions, sliced in ¼-inch
  pieces
½ cup finely chopped Chinese
  cabbage
⅛ head cauliflower, shredded with
  the shredding blade in a food
  processor and then steamed

To make the Egg Fu Yung, beat the egg with half of the soy sauce in a mixing bowl. Measure and reserve ¼ of this mixture for the Fried "Rice" and set aside.

Spray a large wok or skillet with olive oil. Add the ginger, chicken, and vegetables. Stir-fry until the onion is tender. Cool slightly, then add the chicken and vegetables to the egg mixture. Mix well.

Spray the skillet with a little more olive oil. Ladle half of the mixture at a time into the skillet. Fry until the egg is set and both sides are lightly browned. Repeat for the remaining mixture. Set aside.

For the Fried "Rice," spray a large skillet with olive oil. Pour in the reserved egg and cover. Cook undisturbed over medium heat until the egg is set. Set aside.

Add 1 teaspoon olive oil to the wok or skillet. Add the green onions and cabbage. Cook until tender and crisp. Stir in the cauliflower "rice."

Shred the egg and add to the skillet. Add the rest of the soy sauce and mix well. Transfer the Fried "Rice" to a plate and top with the Egg Fu Yung.

Serving Ideas: Serve with green or oolong tea.

> Per Serving: 265 calories; 14 g fat; 21 g protein; 16 g carbohydrate; 4 g dietary fiber; 241 mg cholesterol; 365 mg sodium

Rosemary Grilled Lamb with Goat Cheese, Roasted Beets, Red Onion, and Warm Watercress   (Servings: 1)

Watercress has a slightly bitter taste with a hint of pepper, which is balanced by the sweetness of the roasted beet and red onion. Add the goat cheese, lamb, and the Dijon mustard vinaigrette, and you have flavors that run the full gamut of tastes but blend wonderfully on your taste buds.

1 red onion, sliced
1 teaspoon olive oil
1 large beet, scrubbed, with ends trimmed off
1 lamb chop (trimmed)
salt and pepper to taste
1 garlic clove, crushed

1 teaspoon chopped fresh rosemary
¼ teaspoon Dijon mustard
½ tablespoon white wine vinegar
1 tablespoon extra-virgin olive oil
1 bunch watercress, rinsed and towel dried
1 ounce goat cheese, crumbled

Preheat the oven to 400°. In a bowl, toss the onions in the oil. Spread evenly on one-half of a lightly greased cookie sheet. Place the beet on the other end and roast for 30 minutes or until tender.

Peel the beet and cut it into quarters. Mix the beet and onions together and set aside.

Preheat the grill. Season the lamb chop with the salt, pepper, garlic, and rosemary. Grill for about 5 minutes on each side, or to desired doneness while you make the vinaigrette. Whisk together the mustard, vinegar, salt, and pepper. Add the oil in a stream and blend until emulsified.

In a bowl, toss the beet, onion, watercress, and goat cheese with the vinaigrette. Arrange on a plate and top with the grilled lamb chop.

> Per Serving: 602 calories; 46 g fat; 24 g protein; 24 g carbohydrate; 6 g dietary fiber; 79 mg cholesterol; 235 mg sodium

Lamb Stew (Servings: 2)

1 cup boneless leg of lamb, trimmed of fat and cubed (approximately ½ pound)
1 cup yellow turnips, chopped into 1-inch chunks
1 cup Jerusalem artichokes, scrubbed and chopped into 1-inch chunks

1 cup baby carrots
1 cup chopped yellow onions
2 cups low-sodium beef broth
1 clove garlic, minced
1 teaspoon chopped fresh rosemary
pepper to taste

Heat a heavy stew pot. Add the lamb and caramelize it by cooking it over medium heat until the juices are released and thickened.

Add the remaining ingredients and simmer until the lamb is tender and the vegetables are cooked, about 1 hour.

One serving can be frozen for another meal.

> Per Serving: 327 calories; 6 g fat; 34 g protein; 34 g carbohydrate; 6 g dietary fiber; 62 mg cholesterol; 193 mg sodium

Maui-terranean Salad with Herbed Chicken (Servings: 1)

3 ounces boneless, skinless chicken breast
1 tablespoon lemon juice
1 teaspoon olive oil
½ teaspoon oregano
2 cups mixed baby greens
½ Maui onion or other sweet white onion (e.g., Walla Walla, Vidalia, or Oso)

½ orange, peeled and segmented
5 Kalamata olives, pitted and quartered
⅛ avocado, diced
2 teaspoons extra-virgin olive oil
2 teaspoons red wine vinegar
pepper to taste

Place the chicken breast, lemon juice, 1 teaspoon olive oil, and oregano in a bowl. Cover and marinate for 2 hours.

Grill the chicken. Set aside to cool slightly.

Toss all the remaining ingredients in a salad bowl. Transfer to a serving plate. Slice the chicken breast and place it on top of the salad.

> Per Serving: 371 calories; 21 g fat; 24 g protein; 25 g carbohydrate; 8 g dietary fiber; 49 mg cholesterol; 263 mg sodium

Eggplant Fresh Mozzarella Salad   (Servings: 1)

½ eggplant, sliced in four ½-inch-thick slices
olive oil spray
1 cup arugula
1 teaspoon balsamic vinegar
1 teaspoon extra-virgin olive oil
1 tomato, sliced in four ½-inch-thick slices
2 ounces fresh mozzarella, sliced in four ½-inch-thick slices
8 basil leaves
extra balsamic vinegar for drizzling

Salt the eggplant slices and place them in a strainer. Let them sit for 1 hour, then rinse in water and pat dry with paper towels.

Preheat the oven to 400°.

Spray a baking dish with olive oil and layer with the eggplant. Roast the eggplant for approximately 30 minutes or until it is tender. Set aside to cool.

Toss the arugula with the olive oil and vinegar in a salad bowl. Transfer to a serving plate.

Place the eggplant slices on top of the arugula. Top each with a tomato slice. Place a slice of cheese on top of each stack. Top with two basil leaves. Drizzle with extra vinegar.

> Per Serving: 315 calories; 19 g fat; 16 g protein; 23 g carbohydrate; 7 g dietary fiber; 51 mg cholesterol; 259 mg sodium

Chicken Fajita Salad   (Servings: 1)

olive oil spray
2½ ounces boneless, skinless chicken breast, cut into strips
½ green bell pepper, julienned
½ red bell pepper, julienned
½ onion, julienned
½ teaspoon chili powder
¼ teaspoon cumin
1 cup chopped romaine lettuce
1 cup shredded cabbage
½ cup grape tomatoes
½ cup cooked black beans
½ cup cilantro leaves
juice of ½ lime

Spray a heavy-bottomed pan with olive oil. Heat over medium-high heat. Stir-fry the chicken, peppers, and onions until the chicken is done, approximately 10 minutes. Add the chili powder and the cumin.

Toss the romaine, cabbage, and tomatoes in a salad bowl. Toss the chicken, onions, peppers, and black beans with the ingredients in the salad bowl. Transfer to a plate. Garnish with the cilantro and the lime juice.

> Per Serving: 280 calories; 3 g fat; 28 g protein; 41 g carbohydrate; 13 g dietary fiber; 41 mg cholesterol; 122 mg sodium

Thai Coconut Tempeh   (Servings: 1)

1 stalk lemongrass
3 ounces tempeh, cubed
1 cup zucchini slices
1 small yellow onion, in large dice
1 red bell pepper, in large dice
½ cup coconut milk
½ cup chicken broth

1-inch piece fresh ginger, peeled and thinly sliced
¼ cup basil leaves
½ teaspoon lime zest, or 1 kaffir lime leaf
¼ teaspoon Thai red curry paste

Cut the lemongrass stalk in half and discard the stem. Trim the root end and slice in half lengthwise.

Combine all the ingredients in a saucepan and simmer for approximately 10 minutes or until the vegetables are tender.

Variation: You can substitute 2½ ounces of your favorite protein source for the tempeh.

> Per Serving: 479 calories; 17 g fat; 30 g protein; 62 g carbohydrate; 8 g dietary fiber; 1 mg cholesterol; 58 mg sodium

Chicken Curry   (Servings: 2)

1 tablespoon vegetable oil
½ teaspoon ground turmeric
½ teaspoon ground cumin
½ teaspoon curry powder
½ teaspoon ground ginger
½ teaspoon garam masala
¼ teaspoon pepper

3 cloves garlic, minced
1 medium onion, minced
2 tomatoes, blanched, skinned, and seeded
2 boneless, skinless chicken breast halves, cubed
water

Heat the vegetable oil in a large skillet. Add all the spices. Cook, stirring constantly, until well blended and the aroma is released, about 2 to 3 minutes.

Add the garlic and the onion. Cook on medium heat until the onion is translucent. Add the tomatoes and simmer for approximately 2 minutes or until they are cooked down into a sauce.

Add the chicken and continue simmering until the chicken is done, about 20 minutes. Add the water throughout the cooking process as needed to prevent the curry from becoming dry.

> Per Serving: 245 calories; 9 g fat; 29 g protein; 12 g carbohydrate; 3 g dietary fiber; 68 mg cholesterol; 91 mg sodium

Beef Tenderloin Scalloppini   (Servings: 1)

3 ounces beef tenderloin, pounded to ⅜ inch (scalloppini style)
1 tablespoon olive oil
1 teaspoon finely minced fresh oregano

½ clove garlic, finely minced
pinch of salt and pepper

Combine all the ingredients in a bowl and cover. Marinate for 2 hours in the refrigerator. (This can be done ahead of time.)

Remove the beef and drain the excess oil. Grill for 1 to 2 minutes on each side or until desired doneness.

Serving Ideas: Serve with Broccolini (see the recipe on page 214) and top with Puttanesca Sauce (see the following recipe).

> Per Serving: 251 calories; 19 g fat; 18 g protein; 1 g carbohydrate; trace dietary fiber; 44 mg cholesterol; 41 mg sodium

Puttanesca Sauce   (Servings: 1)

4 roma tomatoes, quartered
2 teaspoons olive oil
olive oil spray
1 clove garlic, chopped
1 teaspoon coarsely chopped black pitted olives

1 teaspoon capers
½ teaspoon minced fresh oregano
1 teaspoon fresh Italian parsley, minced
pinch of red pepper flakes

Preheat the oven to 400°. Toss the tomatoes with the olive oil. Spread on a baking dish sprayed lightly with olive oil. Roast for 20 minutes.

Spray a pan with olive oil. Add the garlic and sauté on medium-high heat for 2 minutes. Add the tomatoes, olives, capers, oregano, parsley, and red pepper flakes. Simmer on medium heat for 10 minutes.

> Per Serving: 192 calories; 11 g fat; 4 g protein; 24 g carbohydrate; 6 g dietary fiber; 0 mg cholesterol; 96 mg sodium

Broccolini (Servings: 1)

6 broccolini spears   juice of half a lemon
1 teaspoon extra-virgin olive oil   salt and pepper to taste

Fill a saucepan with water and bring to a boil. Add the broccolini and cook for 5 minutes. Drain and toss with the olive oil, lemon juice, salt and pepper.

> Per Serving: 41 calories; 5 g fat; trace protein; trace carbohydrate; trace dietary fiber; 0 mg cholesterol; trace sodium

Roast Turkey with Roasted Brussels Sprouts (Servings: 1)

You can roast a half turkey breast, which weighs more than the 3-ounce allowed portion, but it will be more moist than if you roast a smaller amount. After it's roasted, cut off a 3-ounce portion for this dish. The remaining turkey can be frozen in individual portions or used for turkey salad.

3 ounces turkey breast   olive oil spray
8 Brussels sprouts, trimmed

Preheat the oven to 325°. Place the turkey breast half and Brussels sprouts in a roasting pan. Spray the sprouts with the olive oil. Roast for 1 hour or until the turkey's internal temperature is 170° as registered on an instant-read thermometer.

Serving Ideas: Serve with Wild Mushroom Quinoa Dressing (see the following recipe) and Cranberry Apple Compote (see the recipe on page 215).

> Per Serving: 186 calories; 6 g fat; 22 g protein; 14 g carbohydrate; 6 g dietary fiber; 50 mg cholesterol; 83 mg sodium

Wild Mushroom Quinoa Dressing (Servings: 1)

If the mixed mushrooms aren't available, use white or brown button mushrooms.

olive oil spray   ¼ cup chopped celery
½ cup sliced mixed mushrooms, such   ¼ cup quinoa
  as oyster, shiitake, and cremini   ½ cup low-sodium vegetable broth
½ yellow onion, chopped   salt and pepper to taste

Spray a small saucepan with olive oil. Add the mushrooms, onions, and celery and sauté for 2 to 3 minutes over medium-high heat.

Add the quinoa and the vegetable stock, reduce the heat, and simmer until all the liquid is absorbed, approximately 8 to 10 minutes. Season with salt and pepper, if desired.

Per Serving: 218 calories; 3 g fat; 13 g protein; 38 g carbohydrate; 6 g dietary fiber; 0 mg cholesterol; 297 mg sodium

Cranberry Apple Compote (Servings: 1)

¼ cup fresh cranberries
1 large Fuji apple, peeled, cored, and chopped

½ cup water

Combine the cranberries, apple, and water in a small saucepan. Simmer for 8 to 10 minutes.

Per Serving: 246 calories; 1 g fat; 1 g protein; 64 g carbohydrate; 12 g dietary fiber; 0 mg cholesterol; 4 mg sodium

Portobello Mushroom (Servings: 1)

1 large Portobello mushroom cap, whole

olive oil spray

Spray the mushroom cap with olive oil. Grill or roast it in the oven at 350° until tender, approximately 20 minutes.

Per Serving: 31 calories; 1 g fat; 3 g protein; 6 g carbohydrate; 1 g dietary fiber; 0 mg cholesterol; 5 mg sodium

Chicken Cacciatore (Servings: 1)

For a nicely balanced meal, serve the chicken with Portobello Mushroom and Sautéed Swiss Chard.

olive oil spray
1 clove garlic, minced
½ yellow onion, chopped
½ red bell pepper, chopped
3 ounces boneless, skinless chicken breast, cubed
5 roma tomatoes, coarsely chopped in the food processor

1 teaspoon chopped fresh basil
1 teaspoon chopped fresh oregano
1 bay leaf
¼ cup dry red wine
¼ cup low-sodium chicken broth
salt and pepper to taste

Spray a skillet with the olive oil. Sauté the garlic, onion, and pepper over medium heat until the onion is translucent. Add the chicken and simmer for about 5 minutes.

Add the remaining ingredients and simmer over medium-low heat for about 25 minutes.

Note: The red wine can be used during all three steps of the diet because the alcohol is cooked away.

> Per Serving: 320 calories; 3 g fat; 29 g protein; 40 g carbohydrate; 9 g dietary fiber; 49 mg cholesterol; 281 mg sodium

Sautéed Swiss Chard   (Servings: 1)

1 tablespoon olive oil	2 cups Swiss chard
1 clove garlic, minced	salt and pepper to taste

Heat the olive oil in a pan over medium-high heat. Add the garlic and sauté until golden. Add the Swiss chard and sauté for 2 minutes or until tender.

Serving Ideas: Arrange the Swiss chard on a serving plate. Transfer the Portobello Mushroom (see the recipe on page 215) to the Swiss chard and place it top side down. Spoon the Chicken Cacciatore (see the previous recipe) on top of the mushroom.

> Per Serving: 137 calories; 14 g fat; 1 g protein; 4 g carbohydrate; 1 g dietary fiber; 0 mg cholesterol; 154 mg sodium

Lamb Curry   (Servings: 1)

3 teaspoons vegetable oil	1 onion, diced
½ pound boneless leg of lamb, trimmed of fat and cubed	1 clove garlic, minced
½ teaspoon curry powder	½-inch piece fresh ginger, peeled and grated
1 teaspoon dried fenugreek leaves	2 large tomatoes, blanched, peeled, and diced
½ teaspoon ground turmeric	
½ teaspoon garam masala	1 cup water
½ teaspoon ground cumin	salt and pepper to taste
¼ teaspoon red pepper flakes	

Heat 2 teaspoons of the vegetable oil in a large heavy-bottomed pan. Add the lamb and brown over medium-high heat. Remove from the pan and set aside.

Add the remaining teaspoon of oil and turn down the heat to medium. Add all the spices. Cook, stirring constantly, until well blended and the aroma is released, approximately 2 to 3 minutes.

Add the garlic, onion, and ginger and sauté until the onion is translucent. Add the tomatoes and simmer until they are cooked down to a thick sauce.

Add the lamb and the water. Simmer over medium heat for approximately 30 minutes or until the lamb is tender. Season with salt and pepper, if desired.

Serving Ideas: Serve with ½ cup brown rice.

> Per Serving: 282 calories; 13 g fat; 22 g protein; 20 g carbohydrate; 4 g dietary fiber; 59 mg cholesterol; 83 mg sodium

Italian-Style Stuffed Red Bell Pepper   (Servings: 1)

½ cup cooked brown rice
2 teaspoons finely chopped
  onion
1 clove garlic, minced
½ teaspoon Italian seasoning

2 tablespoons tomato sauce
1 egg, slightly beaten
salt and pepper to taste
1 whole red bell pepper, ½ inch
  sliced off top, seeded

Preheat the oven to 350°. Mix the first seven ingredients in a bowl. Stuff the pepper with the mixture.

Spray a small baking dish with the olive oil. Stand the pepper upright in a dish. Bake for 1 hour.

Variation: Substitute leftover barley for the brown rice.

> Per Serving: 233 calories; 6 g fat; 10 g protein; 35 g carbohydrate; 5 g dietary fiber; 212 mg cholesterol; 260 mg sodium

Roasted Vegetable Stew   (Servings: 2)

1 small eggplant, cut into 1-inch cubes
½ pound roma tomatoes, quartered
salt to taste
olive oil spray
3 cloves garlic, minced
1 onion, diced
½ pound mushrooms, quartered
1 red bell pepper, diced

2 zucchini, sliced into ½-inch-thick
  slices
½ pound chopped spinach
1 teaspoon ground cumin
1 tablespoon minced fresh basil
2 tablespoons tahini
juice of ½ lemon

Preheat the oven to 400°. In a large bowl, toss the eggplant and the tomatoes with the salt and olive oil spray to coat well.

Spray the baking dish with olive oil. Spread the eggplant and the tomatoes in the dish. Roast for approximately 30 minutes or until the eggplant begins to brown.

Spray a heavy-bottomed stockpot with olive oil. Over medium heat, sauté the garlic, onion, and mushrooms until the onion pieces are translucent.

Add the red bell pepper and sauté for approximately 2 minutes. Add the eggplant, tomatoes, zucchini, spinach, and spices and simmer for approximately 20 minutes.

Add the tahini and lemon juice. Stir thoroughly to allow the flavors to blend.

Servings Ideas: Serve over ½ cup brown rice. Garnish with toasted pine nuts.

Per Serving: 293 calories; 10 g fat; 15 g protein; 46 g carbohydrate; 17 g dietary fiber; 0 mg cholesterol; 138 mg sodium

Cilantro Shirataki Noodles   (Servings: 1)

(Recipe by Cathy Wong)

3 cups water
1 package shirataki noodles, drained
1 teaspoon olive oil
1 teaspoon minced fresh ginger
1 carrot, grated or sliced into thin matchsticks

¼ cup thinly sliced onion
1 tablespoon rice vinegar
1 teaspoon dark sesame oil
1 teaspoon low-sodium soy sauce
1 tablespoon chopped fresh cilantro

Bring 3 cups of water to a boil in a small pot. Add the noodles and simmer for 3 to 5 minutes. Rinse the noodles with cool water and set aside.

Heat a small pan or skillet on medium heat. Add the olive oil, ginger, carrot, and onion. Sauté until the carrot is tender and the onion is lightly browned.

In a bowl, combine the rice vinegar, sesame oil, soy sauce, and cilantro. Add the sautéed vegetables and noodles and toss. Transfer to a serving plate.

Serving Ideas: Place grilled chicken or beef strips on top of the noodles for a complete meal.

> Per Serving: 156 calories; 9.2 g fat; 1.1 g protein; 17.2 g carbohydrate; 10.5 g dietary fiber; 0 mg cholesterol; 189 mg sodium

Curried Shirataki Noodles   (Servings: 1)

(Recipe by Cathy Wong)

Turmeric or yellow curry powder adds color to the otherwise clear shirataki noodles and a hint of spice.

3 cups water
1 package shirataki noodles, drained
1 teaspoon olive oil
1 clove garlic, minced
1 teaspoon minced fresh ginger
¼ cup thinly sliced red onion
½ teaspoon yellow curry powder (Madras)

½ teaspoon ground turmeric
½ cup thinly sliced napa cabbage
¼ cup very thinly sliced red bell pepper
1½ tablespoons low-fat coconut milk
½ teaspoon low-sodium soy sauce

Bring 3 cups of water to a boil in a small pot. Add the noodles and simmer for 3 to 5 minutes. Rinse the noodles with cool water and set aside.

Heat a small pan or skillet on medium heat. Add the olive oil, garlic, ginger, and onion to the pan and sauté lightly. Add the curry powder and the turmeric and cook for 1 minute. Add the napa cabbage and red bell pepper. Cover the pan and continue cooking until the napa cabbage is wilted. Stir in the coconut milk and soy sauce.

Remove from the heat. Add the noodles and toss the ingredients together. Transfer to a serving plate.

Serving Idea: Serve the noodles with strips of grilled chicken.

> Per Serving: 132 calories; 6.3 g fat; 1.5 g protein; 17.2 g carbohydrate; 11.2 g dietary fiber; 0 mg cholesterol; 99 mg sodium

Snacks, Sauces, Dressings, and Beverages

Jicama Sticks with Roasted Red Pepper-White Bean Dip   (Servings: 4)

Shaped like a turnip but with a light brown skin, jicama (hee-ka-ma) is crunchy, juicy, and sweet like an apple. Eating jicama is a great way to satisfy sweet cravings, because jicama isn't broken down into simple sugars during digestion so it does not elevate blood sugar levels. A cup of cubed jicama is only about 45 calories. It is also a good source of vitamin C and fiber. The peel is inedible and should be discarded. Jicama can be stored in the fridge in a plastic bag for up to two weeks.

1 whole jicama

1 cup canned white beans

1 whole roasted red pepper, peeled and seeded

1 large clove garlic, peeled and crushed

2 teaspoons extra-virgin olive oil

dash freshly ground pepper

Peel the jicama, cut into sticks, and set aside.

Rinse the beans well and drain.

Place the beans and all the remaining ingredients into the bowl of a food processor. Pulse until well blended and smooth. Chill before serving.

> Per Serving: 178 calories; 18 g fat; 2 g protein; 3 g carbohydrate; 1 g dietary fiber; 0 mg cholesterol; 6 mg sodium

Flaxseed Crackers   (Servings: 4)

(Recipe by Cathy Wong)

½ cup ground flaxseeds

1 teaspoon dried basil

1 teaspoon dried oregano

4 cloves garlic, crushed

⅛ teaspoon sea salt

⅛ teaspoon cayenne

½ teaspoon sesame seeds

2 tablespoons water

Preheat the oven to 250°. Lightly spray a cookie sheet with olive oil.

Combine all the ingredients except the water. Once thoroughly mixed, add the water. Place the mixture between two sheets of waxed paper. Use a rolling pin to roll it until it is thin (but it shouldn't be so thin that you can see through it). Gently remove it from both sheets of waxed paper and place it on the cookie sheet. Using a knife, gently cut it into 4 even servings.

Bake the crackers until they are dried thoroughly, approximately 30 to 40 minutes.

> Per Serving: 108 calories; 7 g fat; 4 g protein; 7.3 g carbohydrate; 5.6 g fiber; 0 mg cholesterol; 7 mg sodium

Roasted Cauliflower Florets   (Servings: 8)

(Recipe by Cathy Wong)

4 cups raw cauliflower   sea salt to taste
2 tablespoons olive oil

Preheat the oven to 400°.
Cut the cauliflower into bite-size pieces. Toss in the olive oil and salt.
Place the cauliflower on a baking sheet lined with foil. Bake until the cauliflower is tender and lightly browned, 20 to 35 minutes.

> Per Serving: 45 calories; 3.5 g fat; 1 g protein; 2.6 g carbohydrate; 1.2 g dietary fiber; 0 mg cholesterol; 89 mg sodium

Red Cabbage Live Sauerkraut   (Servings: 6)

(Recipe by Cathy Wong)

1 teaspoon sea salt   ½ cup water
1 teaspoon caraway   ¼ cup fresh lemon juice
1 teaspoon mustard powder   4 cups thinly sliced red cabbage

Mix all the ingredients except the red cabbage in a bowl. Add the cabbage and mix it with the liquid for several minutes. Place the cabbage mixture into a glass jar or container (such as a 4-cup/1-liter Pyrex container). Cover it tightly and let stand for 3 days.

> Per Serving: 9 calories; 10 g fat; 0.3 g protein; 1.7 g carbohydrate; 0.5 g dietary fiber; 0 mg cholesterol; 2 mg sodium

Chickpea Dip   (Servings: 4)

(Recipe by Cathy Wong)

1 can chickpeas   1 teaspoon olive oil
1 clove garlic, crushed   1 tablespoon tahini (sesame seed
2 tablespoons lemon juice   paste)

Rinse the chickpeas well and drain.
Combine all of the ingredients in a blender. Mix until the consistency is smooth.

Serving Ideas: Have ¼ cup of chickpea dip as a midafternoon snack with celery sticks or Flaxseed Crackers (see the recipe on page 220).

> Per Serving: 42 calories; 3.2 g fat; 1 g protein; 2.7 g carbohydrate; 0.5 g dietary fiber; 0 mg cholesterol; 1 mg sodium

Quick Salsa   (Servings: 2)

(Recipe by Cathy Wong)

¼ cup chopped onion   ¼ avocado
2 small tomatoes   ¼ jalapeño pepper
¼ cup cilantro or parsley leaves

   Combine all of the ingredients in a blender. Pulse until everything is finely chopped.

Serving Ideas: Have this salsa as a snack with Flaxseed Crackers (see the recipe on page 220).

> Per Serving: 36 calories; 1.6 g fat; 0.9; g protein; 4.7 g carbohydrate; 1.5 g dietary fiber; 0 mg cholesterol; 9 mg sodium

Cilantro Pesto   (Servings: 4)

(Recipe by Cathy Wong)

This pesto tastes great and is packed with detoxifying nutrients and minerals. The recipe includes Brazil nuts, which are high in the mineral selenium. Limit yourself to one serving of cilantro pesto a day so that you don't exceed the recommended daily intake of selenium.

1 clove garlic   ¼ cup extra-virgin olive oil
½ teaspoon cayenne   1 tablespoon fresh lemon juice
6 Brazil nuts   sea salt to taste
1 cup packed cilantro leaves

   Place all ingredients in a food processor and pulse until smooth.

> Per Serving: 176 calories; 18.3 g fat; 1.2 g protein; 1.8 g carbohydrate; 0.7 g dietary fiber; 0 mg cholesterol; 6 mg sodium

Balsamic Vinaigrette   (Servings: 96)

(Recipe by Cathy Wong)

4 ounces (120 mL) balsamic vinegar   salt and pepper to taste
1 teaspoon mustard   1½ tablespoons minced herbs,
12 ounces (360 mL) extra-virgin olive   such as chives, basil, or parsley
   oil   (optional)

   Combine the vinegar and the mustard. Gradually whisk in the oil. Add salt and pepper, if desired. If using herbs, mix them in.

> Per Serving: 30 calories; 3.4 g fat; 0 g protein; 0.1 g carbohydrate; 0 g dietary fiber; 0 mg cholesterol; 0 mg sodium

Cleansing Lemon Tea   (Servings: 1)

(Recipe by Cathy Wong)

1 slice of organic lemon (peel included)

cinnamon stick

1 rooibos teabag or 1 teaspoon loose leaves

stevia or other allowed sweetener (optional)

Place the cinnamon stick into a mug with the lemon slice and rooibos teabag. Pour hot water into the mug and allow the tea to steep for 3 minutes, covered. Remove the teabag and continue to steep for 7 minutes. Sweeten with the stevia if desired.

> Per Serving: 5 calories; 0 g fat; 0.1 g protein; 1.2 g carbohydrate; 0.5 g dietary fiber; 0 mg cholesterol; 0 mg sodium

Desserts

Carob Mac Nut Drops   (Servings: 40)

1 cup carob chips

½ cup almond butter

1 teaspoon vanilla extract

¾ teaspoon chopped macadamia nuts

½ cup dried cranberries

Melt the carob chips and the almond butter in a double boiler. Stir continuously. Remove from the heat when the almond butter and the carob are well blended but there are still little bits of chips that haven't melted.

Add the vanilla, nuts, and cranberries. Mix well.

Drop rounded tablespoons of the mixture onto a cookie sheet lined with waxed paper. Place in the refrigerator until the drops are set.

Variation: Substitute raisins for the cranberries. Dark chocolate chips can be substituted for the carob chips. You can also substitute another nut butter for the almond butter.

> Per Serving: 70 calories; 6 g fat; 1 g protein; 4 g carbohydrate; 1 g dietary fiber; trace cholesterol; 7 mg sodium

Lemon Cream with Raspberries   (Servings: 1)

(Recipe by Cathy Wong)

⅓ cup low-fat coconut milk

¼ teaspoon organic lemon extract

¼ teaspoon organic pure vanilla extract

¼ teaspoon grated lemon rind

2½ teaspoons lecithin granules

½ cup organic raspberries

Place the coconut milk in the blender with the lemon extract, vanilla extract, and lemon rind. Add the lecithin granules (available at health food stores). Blend until smooth and creamy. Pour into a small serving bowl and top with the raspberries.

Per Serving: 126 calories; 11.3 g fat; 0.3 g protein; 5.8 g carbohydrate; 2.2 g dietary fiber; 0 mg cholesterol; 16 mg sodium

Pomegranate Poached Pear (Servings: 1)

(Recipe by Cathy Wong)

1 Bosc pear
1 cup unsweetened pomegranate
  juice
¼ teaspoon ground nutmeg

1 cinnamon stick
½ teaspoon vanilla extract
½ tablespoon pomegranate seeds
  (optional)

Peel the pear, leaving on the stem, and slice in half lengthwise. Remove the core. Mix the juice, nutmeg, cinnamon, and vanilla in a small saucepan. Bring to a simmer. Place the pear halves in the liquid and poach for approximately 15 minutes, or until very tender, turning the pear halves over halfway through cooking.

Remove the pear halves from the liquid and place them upright in a small serving bowl. Spoon 2 teaspoons of the poaching liquid around the pears. Garnish with pomegranate seeds, if using. Serve immediately.

Variation: Top with ¼ cup of nonfat vanilla yogurt mixed with a dash of ground cinnamon.

Per Serving: 140 calories; 0.8 g fat; 0.6 g protein; 32.6 g carbohydrate; 4.1 g dietary fiber; 0 mg cholesterol; 2 mg sodium

Blueberry Granola Crisp (Servings: 2)

(Recipe by Cathy Wong)

1½ cups fresh blueberries
½ teaspoon vanilla extract

1½ tablespoons Flaxseed Granola
  (see recipe on page 196)

Preheat the oven to 400°.

Combine the blueberries and the vanilla in a bowl. Divide the blueberry mixture in half and place each half in a ramekin. Top with the granola.

Place the ramekins on a baking sheet. Bake until the tops appear bubbly and golden brown, 15 to 20 minutes. Remove from the oven and serve hot.

Serving Ideas: Place a dollop of nonfat frozen yogurt on top of the blueberry crisp before serving.

> Per Serving: 212 calories; 5 g fat; 3.8 g protein; 38.3 g carbohydrate; 7.8 g dietary fiber; 0 mg cholesterol; 25 mg sodium

Dark Chocolate Dipped Strawberries   (Servings: 4)

(Recipe by Cathy Wong)

1 pound (16 ounces) whole   2 ounces dark chocolate
  strawberries

Wash the strawberries thoroughly, keeping the green tops on, and pat them until they are completely dry.

Place the chocolate in a small bowl or dish and microwave it for 30 seconds. If the chocolate isn't yet melted, continue microwaving for 10 seconds at a time until it is melted. Remove the chocolate from the microwave.

Prepare a baking sheet lined with waxed paper. Dip each strawberry in the melted chocolate, covering the lower portion of each with a thin layer of chocolate. Place each one on the waxed paper.

Place the baking sheet in the refrigerator until the chocolate hardens. Divide into four even portions and place in serving dishes.

> Per Serving: 117 calories; 5 g fat; 1.4 g protein; 16.6 g carbohydrate; 3.3 g dietary fiber; 0 mg cholesterol; 2 mg sodium

Microwave Apple Crumble   (Servings: 1)

(Recipe by Cathy Wong)

1 tablespoon chopped walnuts   ½ teaspoon brown sugar or rapadura
1 teaspoon ground flaxseeds   1 apple (e.g., Northern Spy, Rome
¼ teaspoon ground cinnamon   Beauty, York Imperial, Gala)

Preheat the oven to 300°.

Combine all of the ingredients except the apple in a bowl and spread the mixture on a foil-lined baking sheet. Bake the mixture in the oven until lightly browned, about 5 minutes.

Peel and core the apple. Place it in a covered microwave-safe bowl and microwave the apple for 2 to 2½ minutes or until it is warm and tender.

Place the apple in a serving dish and top with the baked mixture. Serve immediately.

Serving Ideas: Top the apple with ¼ cup of cold nonfat vanilla yogurt (or frozen yogurt) mixed with a dash of cinnamon.

> Per Serving: 186 calories; 6.4 g fat; 2.2 g protein; 29.7 g carbohydrate; 6.4 g dietary fiber; 0 mg cholesterol; 5 mg sodium

Pomegranate Popsicles   (Servings: 6)

(Recipe by Cathy Wong)

2 cups vanilla nonfat yogurt
1 cup unsweetened pomegranate
  juice

Mix together the yogurt and the pomegranate juice until fully combined. Pour into six popsicle molds and freeze.

> Per Serving: 72 calories; 0.2 g fat; 4.7 g protein; 12.7 g carbohydrate; 0.1 g dietary fiber; 1 mg cholesterol; 64 mg sodium

Appendix

The 28-Day Meal Plan

1,200 Calories a Day

Capital letters indicate that the recipe is included in this book.

Day 1

Breakfast	Muesli Cereal and Cleansing Lemon Tea
Lunch	Maui-terranean Salad with Herbed Chicken and green tea
Midafternoon Snack	¾ cup blackberries topped with 1 teaspoon toasted ground flaxseeds
Dinner	Roast Turkey with Roasted Brussels Sprouts and Cranberry Apple Compote

Day 2

Breakfast	Asparagus Frittata and green tea
Midmorning Snack	Fruit Salad with Orange Mint Dressing
Lunch	Super Green Chicken Soup, salad (1 cup mixed greens, 1 cup arugula, diced red peppers, 1 diced roma tomato) with 1 tablespoon Balsamic Vinaigrette and 1 teaspoon ground flaxseeds
Midafternoon Snack	Cleansing Lemon Tea and apple with 10 almonds
Dinner	grilled wild salmon, steamed broccolini, broccoli, or bok choy, and ½ cup brown rice mixed with 2 teaspoons flaxseeds
Dessert	Carob Mac Nut Drop

Day 3

Breakfast	Blueberry Flax Cereal
Lunch	Sweet Potato with Curried Vegetables and Watercress and Leek Soup
Midafternoon Snack	Jicama Sticks with Roasted Red Pepper-White Bean Dip

Dinner	Chicken Stir-Fry over "Rice"
Dessert	Pomegranate Poached Pear and Cleansing Lemon Tea

Day 4

Breakfast	Raspberry Almond Smoothie
Lunch	Black-Eyed Pea Stew, Arugula Salad, and 1 teaspoon ground flaxseeds
Midafternoon Snack	apple and Cleansing Lemon Tea
Dinner	Grilled Chicken Breast with Roasted Vegetable Salsa served on Zucchini Medley and 1 teaspoon ground flaxseeds
Dessert	¼ cup berries with 1 teaspoon ground flaxseeds

Day 5

Breakfast	Candied Sweet Potato and Cleansing Lemon Tea
Lunch	Thai Coconut Tempeh and 1 teaspoon ground flaxseeds
Midafternoon Snack	¾ cup blueberries topped with 1 teaspoon toasted ground flaxseeds
Dinner	Brown Rice with Kale, Vegetarian Chili, and 1 teaspoon ground flaxseeds
Dessert	Carob Mac Nut Drop

Day 6

Breakfast	Pumpkin Pie Oatmeal
Midmorning Snack	½ cup cherries topped with 1 teaspoon sliced almonds and Cleansing Lemon Tea
Lunch	Chicken Fajita Salad and an apple
Midafternoon Snack	Flaxseed Crackers with Quick Salsa
Dinner	Grilled Turkey Breast Cutlet, Mixed Baby Greens with Blood Oranges, Almonds, and Pomegranates, steamed asparagus, and ½ cup quinoa
Dessert	Lemon Cream with Raspberries

Day 7

Breakfast	2 Southwestern Egg Cups
Midmorning Snack	¾ cup berries topped with 2 teaspoons toasted ground flaxseeds and 1 tablespoon sliced almonds
Lunch	Watercress and Leek Soup and Sweet Potato with Curried Vegetables
Midafternoon Snack	raw vegetables with 2 tablespoons Chickpea Dip and Cleansing Lemon Tea
Dinner	Black Bean and Pumpkin Soup with Chicken, Arugula Salad, and 1 teaspoon ground flaxseeds

Day 8

Breakfast	Two-Minute Omelet and 1 teaspoon toasted ground flaxseeds
Midmorning Snack	½ cup organic low-fat yogurt or kefir (test food)
Lunch	Brussels Sprouts Soup and sliced grilled chicken on 2 cups baby greens with sliced beets, shaved red onion, and diced tomatoes with 1 tablespoon Balsamic Vinaigrette
Midafternoon Snack	½ cup Roasted Cauliflower Florets with 2 tablespoons Chickpea Dip and Cleansing Lemon Tea
Dinner	Grilled Turkey Breast Cutlet, Mixed Baby Greens with Blood Oranges, Almonds, and Pomegranates, and 2 teaspoons ground flaxseeds
Dessert	pear

Day 9

Breakfast	2 Southwestern Egg Cups and 1 teaspoon ground flaxseeds
Midmorning Snack	cheese (any type of low-fat hard cheese), 1 ounce (test food)
Lunch	Super Green Chicken Soup and small sweet potato
Midafternoon Snack	apple and Cleansing Lemon Tea
Dinner	Chicken Curry, Roasted Cauliflower Florets, steamed spinach, and 2 teaspoons ground flaxseeds
Dessert	¾ cup strawberries with 1 tablespoon sliced almonds

Day 10

Breakfast	Blueberry Flax Cereal
Midmorning Snack	Barley, ½ cup (test food)
Lunch	Roasted Vegetable Stew, ½ cup brown rice mixed with 1 teaspoon flaxseeds, and ¼ cup raw broccoli sprouts or ½ cup steamed broccoli or broccolini
Dinner	Chicken Stir-fry over "Rice"
Dessert	apple and Cleansing Lemon Tea

Day 11

Breakfast	Two-Minute Omelet
Midmorning Snack	whole wheat spaghetti, ½ cup cooked (test food)
Lunch	Chicken Fajita Salad and 1 teaspoon ground flaxseeds
Midafternoon Snack	raw vegetables with 2 tablespoons Chickpea Dip and Cleansing Lemon Tea
Dinner	Grilled Chicken Breast, salad (1 cup arugula, 1 cup mixed greens, ¾ cup beets, thinly sliced red onions, grape tomatoes, 1 tablespoon crushed walnuts, black olives) with 1 tablespoon Balsamic Vinaigrette, ½ cup cooked quinoa, and 2 teaspoons ground flaxseeds
Dessert	Carob Mac Nut Drop

Day 12

Breakfast	Raspberry Almond Smoothie
Midmorning Snack	1 slice rye bread (test food)
Lunch	Roasted Vegetable Stew, ½ cup brown rice with 1 teaspoon ground flaxseeds, salad (1 cup mixed greens, 1 cup arugula, diced red peppers, and 1 roma tomato, diced) with 1 tablespoon Balsamic Vinaigrette
Midafternoon Snack	apple and Cleansing Lemon Tea
Dinner	Grilled Turkey Breast Cutlet, ½ cup Red Cabbage Live Sauerkraut, ½ cup cooked quinoa, and 2 teaspoons ground flaxseeds

Day 13

Breakfast	Pumpkin Pie Oatmeal
Midmorning Snack	1 cup skim milk (test food)
Lunch	Maui-terranean Salad with Herbed Chicken and 2 teaspoons toasted ground flaxseeds
Midafternoon Snack	½ cup berries with 1 teaspoon toasted ground flaxseeds and Cleansing Lemon Tea
Dinner	3 ounces roasted turkey breast, Cranberry Apple Compote, and Arugula Salad

Day 14

Breakfast	Eggs Florentine
Midmorning Snack	1 slice whole grain bread (test food)
Lunch	Chicken Curry, Chopped Salad, and 2 teaspoons ground flaxseeds
Midafternoon Snack	pear slices with 1 tablespoon almond butter, 1 teaspoon ground flaxseeds, and Cleansing Lemon Tea
Dinner	Chicken Egg Fu Yung with Fried "Rice"

Day 15

Breakfast	Candied Sweet Potato
Midafternoon Snack	¾ cup berries, ½ cup low-fat yogurt, and 1 teaspoon toasted ground flaxseeds
Lunch	Curried Chicken Salad in Lettuce Wrap
Midafternoon Snack	apple and Cleansing Lemon Tea
Dinner	Portobello Mushroom with Chicken Cacciatore on Sautéed Swiss Chard and 2 teaspoons ground flaxseeds

Day 16

Breakfast	Cherry Kefir Smoothie and Cleansing Lemon Tea
Lunch	Barley-Lentil Soup with Swiss Chard, Chopped Salad, and 1 teaspoon ground flaxseeds
Midafternoon Snack	roasted cauliflower and 2 tablespoons Chickpea Dip

Dinner	Beef Tenderloin Scaloppini, Puttanesca Sauce, Broccolini, and 2 teaspoons ground flaxseeds
Dessert	¼ cup berries

Day 17

Breakfast	¾ cup berries, ½ cup low-fat yogurt, 2 teaspoons toasted ground flaxseeds, and 1 tablespoon protein powder
Midmorning Snack	1 slice bread (e.g., rye) with tomato slices drizzled with ½ teaspoon olive oil and balsamic vinegar
Lunch	Brussels Sprouts Soup with sliced Grilled Chicken Breast, Italian flat-leaf parsley, thin shavings of parmesan, ½ cup chickpeas, ⅓ cup quinoa, and 1 tablespoon lemon-olive oil vinaigrette
Midafternoon Snack	⅓ cup unsweetened applesauce with 1 tablespoon sliced almonds, 1 teaspoon toasted ground flaxseeds, and ground cinnamon
Dinner	Rosemary Grilled Lamb with Goat Cheese, Roasted Beets and Red Onion with Warm Watercress

Day 18

Breakfast	Scrambled Egg Oatmeal
Lunch	Chicken Fajita Salad
Midafternoon Snack	blackberries with 1 teaspoon ground flaxseeds and ½ cup low-fat yogurt
Dinner	wild salmon, steamed asparagus, artichoke, ½ cup brown rice, 2 teaspoons ground flaxseeds
Dessert	Carob Mac Nut Drop

Day 19

Breakfast	Eggs Florentine
Midmorning Snack	apple with 10 almonds
Lunch	Chicken Egg Fu Yung with Fried "Rice" and 1 teaspoon ground flaxseeds
Midafternoon Snack	Jicama Sticks with Roasted Red Pepper-White Bean Dip
Dinner	Grilled Beef Tenderloin Salad, Watercress and Leek Soup, and 2 teaspoons ground flaxseeds

Day 20

Breakfast	Berry Smoothie
Lunch	Curried Chicken Salad in Lettuce Wrap, red and green pepper strips, and sliced cucumbers
Midafternoon Snack	raw vegetables, Flaxseed Crackers or ½ (six ½ inch) whole wheat pita with 2 tablespoons Chickpea Dip
Dinner	Roast Turkey with Roasted Brussels Sprouts, Wild Mushroom Quinoa Dressing, and Cranberry Apple Compote

Day 21

Breakfast	Pumpkin Pie Oatmeal
Lunch	Eggplant Fresh Mozzarella Salad and sliced Grilled Chicken Breast
Midafternoon Snack	¾ cup berries with flaxseeds
Dinner	Lamb Stew, ½ cup quinoa, and flaxseeds

Day 22

Breakfast	Blueberry Flax Cereal
Midmorning Snack	apple
Lunch	Italian-Style Stuffed Red Bell Pepper and Arugula Salad
Midafternoon Snack	Flaxseed Crackers or ½ whole wheat pita with 2 tablespoons Chickpea Dip
Dinner	Brown Rice with Kale, Vegetarian Chili

Day 23

Breakfast	Scrambled Egg Oatmeal
Midmorning Snack	pear with 7 walnut halves
Lunch	Black Bean and Pumpkin Soup with Chicken
Midafternoon Snack	roasted cauliflower with 2 tablespoons Chickpea Dip and Flaxseed Crackers or ½ whole wheat pita
Dinner	4-ounce tilapia fillet, steamed spinach, steamed bok choy or other cruciferous vegetable, ½ cup quinoa, and flaxseeds

Day 24

Breakfast	Cherry Kefir Smoothie
Midmorning Snack	apple
Lunch	Black-Eyed Pea Stew
Midafternoon Snack	jicama sticks sprinkled with lime juice
Dinner	Grilled Chicken Breast, Roasted Vegetable Salsa, and Zucchini Medley
Dessert	½ cup berries with sliced almonds

Day 25

Breakfast	Berry Smoothie
Lunch	3 ounces sliced Grilled Chicken Breast, artichokes with vinaigrette, ½ cup cooked barley, Broccolini, and flaxseeds
Dinner	Portobello Mushroom with Chicken Cacciatore on Sautéed Swiss Chard and flaxseeds

Day 26

Breakfast	1 soft-boiled egg, 1 slice turkey bacon, tomato slices, and 1 slice bread (e.g., rye)
Midmorning Snack	¾ cup berries topped with flaxseeds
Lunch	Barley-Lentil Soup with Swiss Chard and Chopped Salad
Midafternoon Snack	½ cup roasted cauliflower
Dinner	Thai Coconut Tempeh

Day 27

Breakfast	Pumpkin Pie Oatmeal
Lunch	Jerusalem Artichoke and Leek Soup, Arugula Salad with ¾ cup beets, black olives, and lemon-olive oil vinaigrette topped with 1 ounce feta or low-fat goat cheese, and flaxseeds
Midafternoon Snack	2 tablespoons Chickpea Dip, black olives, and Flaxseed Crackers or pita wedges (half a 6½ inch-diameter pita)
Dinner	Lamb Curry, spaghetti squash, and flaxseeds

Day 28

Breakfast	Berry Smoothie
Midmorning Snack	1 slice rye bread with tomato slices drizzled with ½ teaspoon olive oil and balsamic vinegar
Lunch	3 ounces sliced Grilled Chicken Breast, artichokes with vinaigrette, ½ cup cooked barley, Broccolini, and flaxseeds
Dinner	Chicken Stir-Fry over "Rice"

1,800 Calories a Day

Day 1

Breakfast	Muesli Cereal (use ½ cup blackberries)
Midmorning Snack	apple with 10 almonds and Cleansing Lemon Tea
Lunch	Maui-terranean Salad with Herbed Chicken, Jerusalem Artichoke and Leek Soup, ½ cup cooked quinoa
Midafternoon Snack	¾ cup strawberries topped with 1 teaspoon toasted flaxseeds
Dinner	Roast Turkey with Roasted Brussels Sprouts, Wild Mushroom Quinoa Dressing, and Cranberry Apple Compote

Day 2

Breakfast	Asparagus Frittata and 2 slices turkey bacon
Midmorning Snack	Fruit Salad with Orange Mint Dressing
Lunch	Super Green Chicken Soup, salad (1 cup mixed greens, 1 cup arugula, diced red peppers, and 1 diced roma tomato), with 1 tablespoon Balsamic Vinaigrette, 1 teaspoon ground flaxseeds, and ½ cup cooked quinoa
Midafternoon Snack	apple with 10 almonds and Cleansing Lemon Tea
Dinner	4 ounces wild salmon grilled with 1 teaspoon olive oil, steamed broccolini, broccoli, or bok choy with 1 teaspoon olive oil and low-sodium soy sauce or tamari, and ½ cup brown rice mixed with 2 teaspoons flaxseeds
Dessert	Carob Mac Nut Drop

Day 3

Breakfast	Blueberry Flax Cereal
Midmorning Snack	apple and 12 almonds and Cleansing Lemon Tea
Lunch	3-ounce Grilled Chicken Breast, Sweet Potato with Curried Vegetables, and Watercress and Leek Soup
Midafternoon Snack	Jicama Sticks with Roasted Red Pepper–White Bean Dip
Dinner	Chicken Stir-Fry over "Rice," 1 cup steamed spinach or green beans, and ½ cup cooked brown rice or quinoa
Dessert	Pomegranate Poached Pear

Day 4

Breakfast	Raspberry Almond Smoothie
Midmorning Snack	apple with 5 almonds and Cleansing Lemon Tea
Lunch	Black-Eyed Pea Stew, Arugula Salad, and 1 teaspoon ground flaxseeds
Midafternoon Snack	raw vegetables with 2 tablespoons Chickpea Dip
Dinner	Grilled Chicken Breast with Roasted Vegetable Salsa served with Zucchini Medley and 1 teaspoon ground flaxseeds
Dessert	½ cup berries with 1 teaspoon ground flaxseeds

Day 5

Breakfast	Candied Sweet Potato
Midmorning Snack	pear with 7 walnut halves and Cleansing Lemon Tea
Lunch	Thai Coconut Tempeh, 1 teaspoon ground flaxseeds, and ½ cup cooked brown rice
Midafternoon Snack	¾ cup blueberries topped with 1 tablespoon sliced almonds
Dinner	Brown Rice with Kale, Vegetarian Chili, 3 ounces Grilled Chicken Breast, and 2 teaspoons ground flaxseeds
Dessert	Carob Mac Nut Drop

Day 6

Breakfast	Pumpkin Pie Oatmeal
Midmorning Snack	1 cup berries topped with 1 tablespoon sliced almonds
Lunch	Chicken Fajita Salad, ½ cup quinoa mixed with 1 teaspoon ground flaxseeds, ¼ avocado, pear, and Cleansing Lemon Tea
Midafternoon Snack	1 cup Roasted Cauliflower Florets with 5 black olives and 2 tablespoons Chickpea Dip
Dinner	4 ounces Grilled Turkey Breast Cutlet, Mixed Baby Greens with Blood Oranges, Almonds, and Pomegranates, ½ cup cooked brown rice, and 2 teaspoon flaxseeds
Dessert	Lemon Cream with Raspberries

Day 7

Breakfast	3 Southwestern Egg Cups and Cleansing Lemon Tea
Midmorning Snack	1 cup berries topped with 1 tablespoon sliced almonds
Lunch	3 ounces grilled bison, Watercress and Leek Soup, and Sweet Potato with Curried Vegetables
Midafternoon Snack	raw vegetables with 2 tablespoons Chickpea Dip and 6 black olives
Dinner	Black Bean and Pumpkin Soup with Chicken, Arugula Salad, and ½ cup cooked quinoa
Dessert	Microwave Apple Crumble

Day 8

Breakfast	Two-Minute Omelet (portions: 3 egg whites, 2 tablespoons low-fat coconut milk, and 2 slices turkey bacon)
Midmorning Snack	½ cup organic low-fat yogurt or kefir (test food)
Lunch	Brussels Sprouts Soup, 4 ounces sliced grilled beef on 2 cups baby greens with ¾ cup sliced beets, shaved red onion, and diced tomatoes with 1 tablespoon Balsamic Vinaigrette, 1 teaspoon ground flaxseeds, 1 small sweet potato, and ½ cup cooked brown rice or quinoa
Midafternoon Snack	1 cup Roasted Cauliflower Florets and 2 tablespoons Chickpea Dip
Dinner	Grilled Turkey Breast Cutlet, Mixed Baby Greens with Blood Oranges, Almonds, and Pomegranates, ½ cup cooked quinoa, and 2 teaspoons ground flaxseeds
Dessert	Pomegranate Poached Pear and Cleansing Lemon Tea

Day 9

Breakfast	3 Southwestern Egg Cups and 1 teaspoon ground flaxseeds
Midmorning Snack	cheese (any type of low-fat cheese), 1 ounce (test food)
Lunch	Super Green Chicken Soup, Candied Sweet Potato, salad (1 cup mixed greens, 1 cup arugula, diced red peppers, and 1 diced roma tomato) with 1 tablespoon Balsamic Vinaigrette

Midafternoon Snack	pear with 7 walnut halves and Cleansing Lemon Tea
Dinner	Chicken Curry, Roasted Cauliflower Florets, steamed spinach, and ½ cup cooked brown rice mixed with 2 teaspoons ground flaxseeds
Dessert	¾ cup strawberries with 1 tablespoon sliced almonds

Day 10

Breakfast	Blueberry Flax Cereal (use ¾ cup almond milk)
Midmorning Snack	barley, ½ cup cooked (test food)
Lunch	Roasted Vegetable Stew, ¼ cup broccoli sprouts or ½ cup steamed broccoli or broccolini, ½ cup cooked brown rice, and 4 ounces Grilled Chicken Breast
Midafternoon Snack	raw vegetables with 2 tablespoons Chickpea Dip
Dinner	Chicken Stir-Fry over "Rice" and steamed green beans or spinach
Dessert	apple with 12 almonds and Cleansing Lemon Tea

Day 11

Breakfast	Two-Minute Omelet (portions: 3 egg whites, 2 tablespoons low-fat coconut milk, and 2 slices turkey bacon) and Cleansing Lemon Tea
Midmorning Snack	whole wheat spaghetti, ½ cup cooked (test food)
Lunch	Chicken Fajita Salad, 1 teaspoon flaxseeds, ½ cup cooked quinoa, ¼ avocado, and a pear
Midafternoon Snack	raw vegetables and 2 tablespoons Chickpea Dip
Dinner	4 ounces Grilled Chicken Breast, salad (1 cup arugula, 1 cup mixed greens, ¾ cup beets, thinly sliced red onions, grape tomatoes, 1 tablespoon crushed walnuts, 5 black olives) with 1 tablespoon Balsamic Vinaigrette, 2 teaspoons ground flaxseeds, and ½ cup cooked brown rice
Dessert	Carob Mac Nut Drop

Day 12

Breakfast	Raspberry Almond Smoothie
Midmorning Snack	1 slice rye bread (test food)
Lunch	4 ounces grilled beef, Roasted Vegetable Stew, ½ cup cooked brown rice with 1 teaspoon ground flaxseeds, salad (1 cup mixed greens, 1 cup arugula, diced red peppers, 1 diced roma tomato) with 1 tablespoon Balsamic Vinaigrette
Midafternoon Snack	apple with 12 almonds and Cleansing Lemon Tea
Dinner	Grilled Turkey Breast Cutlet, ½ cup Red Cabbage Live Sauerkraut with 1 tablespoon Balsamic Vinaigrette, steamed spinach, and ½ cup cooked brown rice with 1 tablespoon ground flaxseeds

Day 13

Breakfast	Pumpkin Pie Oatmeal
Midmorning Snack	1 cup skim milk (test food)
Lunch	Maui-terranean Salad with Herbed Chicken, ½ cup cooked quinoa, and 2 teaspoons ground flaxseeds
Midafternoon Snack	½ cup berries and 1 teaspoon toasted ground flaxseeds
Dinner	4 ounces roasted turkey breast, Cranberry Apple Compote, and Arugula Salad
Dessert	apple and Cleansing Lemon Tea

Day 14

Breakfast	Eggs Florentine and 2 turkey breakfast links
Midmorning Snack	1 slice whole grain bread (test food)
Lunch	Chicken Curry, Chopped Salad, ½ cup brown rice with 2 teaspoons ground flaxseeds
Midafternoon Snack	pear slices with 1½ tablespoons almond butter, 1 teaspoon ground flaxseeds, and Cleansing Lemon Tea
Dinner	Chicken Egg Fu Yung with Fried "Rice," steamed spinach or green beans, and ½ cup cooked barley
Dessert	1 cup berries and 1 cup low-fat yogurt

Day 15

Breakfast	Candied Sweet Potato
Midmorning Snack	¾ cup berries, ½ cup low-fat yogurt, 1 tablespoon vanilla protein powder, and 1 teaspoon toasted ground flaxseeds
Lunch	Curried Chicken Salad in Lettuce Wrap, red and green pepper strips, sliced cucumbers, Cleansing Lemon Tea, and apple with 10 almonds
Midafternoon Snack	1 cup Roasted Cauliflower Florets with 5 black olives and 2 tablespoons Chickpea Dip
Dinner	Portobello Mushroom with Chicken Cacciatore on Sautéed Swiss Chard, 2 teaspoons ground flaxseeds, and ½ cup cooked barley

Day 16

Breakfast	Cherry Kefir Smoothie
Midmorning Snack	pear with 10 almonds
Lunch	Barley-Lentil Soup with Swiss Chard, Chopped Salad, 1 teaspoon ground flaxseeds, and 1 slice bread (e.g., whole grain, rye)
Midafternoon Snack	raw vegetables and 2 tablespoons Chickpea Dip
Dinner	Beef Tenderloin Scalloppini with Puttanesca Sauce and Broccolini, ½ cup cooked barley, and 2 teaspoons ground flaxseeds
Dessert	Dark Chocolate Dipped Strawberries

Day 17

Breakfast	¾ cup berries with ¾ cup low-fat yogurt, 2 teaspoons toasted ground flaxseeds, and 2 teaspoons protein powder
Midmorning Snack	1 slice bread with tomato slices drizzled with ½ teaspoon olive oil and balsamic vinegar topped with 1 ounce goat cheese
Lunch	Brussels Sprouts Soup, sliced Grilled Chicken Breast with Italian flat-leaf parsley, thin shavings of parmesan, ½ cup chickpeas, and 1 tablespoon lemon-olive oil vinaigrette, and ½ cup cooked quinoa
Midafternoon Snack	Microwave Apple Crumble
Dinner	Rosemary Grilled Lamb with Goat Cheese, Roasted Beets, Red Onion, and Warm Watercress, 1 teaspoon ground flaxseeds, ½ cup cooked quinoa, brown rice, or barley, and Cleansing Lemon Tea

Day 18

Breakfast	Scrambled Egg Oatmeal
Midmorning Snack	pear with 7 walnut halves and Cleansing Lemon Tea
Lunch	Chicken Fajita Salad, ½ cup cooked quinoa, 1 teaspoon ground flaxseeds, and ¼ avocado
Midafternoon Snack	¾ cup blackberries, 1 teaspoon ground flaxseeds, and 1 cup low-fat yogurt
Dinner	wild salmon grilled with 1 teaspoon olive oil, steamed asparagus, ¾ cup artichokes with 1 tablespoon lemon-olive oil vinaigrette, and 1 teaspoon ground flaxseeds
Dessert	Carob Mac Nut Drop

Day 19

Breakfast	Eggs Florentine and 2 turkey breakfast links
Midmorning Snack	apple with 10 almonds
Lunch	Chicken Egg Fu Yung with Fried "Rice," steamed spinach or green beans, ½ cup cooked barley, and 1 teaspoon ground flaxseeds
Midafternoon Snack	Jicama Sticks with Roasted Red Pepper-White Bean Dip
Dinner	Grilled Beef Tenderloin Salad, Watercress and Leek Soup, and ½ cup cooked barley
Dessert	½ cup berries, ½ cup low-fat yogurt, and Cleansing Lemon Tea

Day 20

Breakfast	Berry Smoothie
Midmorning Snack	pear with 10 almonds
Lunch	Curried Chicken Salad in Lettuce Wrap, red and green pepper strips, and sliced cucumbers

Midafternoon Snack	raw vegetables with 2 tablespoons Chickpea Dip and 5 black olives, one 6½-inch warmed whole wheat pita, and 1 teaspoon ground flaxseeds
Dinner	Roast Turkey with Roasted Brussels Sprouts, Wild Mushroom Quinoa Dressing, Cranberry Apple Compote, and 2 teaspoons ground flaxseeds

Day 21

Breakfast	Pumpkin Pie Oatmeal
Midafternoon Snack	¾ cup berries, 1 teaspoon ground flaxseeds, and ¾ cup low-fat yogurt or kefir mixed with 2 teaspoons whey protein powder
Lunch	Eggplant Fresh Mozzarella Salad, 3 ounces sliced Grilled Chicken Breast, ½ cup cooked barley, and Cleansing Lemon Tea
Midafternoon Snack	pear with 7 walnut halves
Dinner	Lamb Stew, 2 teaspoons ground flaxseeds, and ½ cup cooked quinoa

Day 22

Breakfast	Blueberry Flax Cereal (use ¾ cup almond milk)
Midmorning Snack	apple with 12 almonds and Cleansing Lemon Tea
Lunch	Italian-Style Stuffed Red Bell Pepper, Arugula Salad, and 3 ounces grilled beef
Midafternoon Snack	Flaxseed Crackers and 2 tablespoons Chickpea Dip
Dinner	4 ounces Grilled Chicken Breast, Brown Rice with Kale, and Vegetarian Chili

Day 23

Breakfast	Scrambled Egg Oatmeal, 1 cup berries, and ½ cup kefir
Midmorning Snack	pear with 7 walnut halves
Lunch	Black Bean and Pumpkin Soup with Chicken and 1 slice bread, open-faced, topped with sliced tomatoes, cheese, sprouts, and 1 teaspoon ground flaxseeds
Midafternoon Snack	Roasted Cauliflower Florets with 2 tablespoons Chickpea Dip
Dinner	4 ounces grilled tilapia fillet with 2 teaspoons olive oil, ½ cup steamed spinach, ½ cup steamed bok choy or other cruciferous vegetable, ½ cup cooked barley, and 2 teaspoons ground flaxseeds

Day 24

Breakfast	Cherry Kefir Smoothie
Midmorning Snack	apple with 12 almonds

Lunch	Black-Eyed Pea Stew, 2 teaspoons ground flaxseeds, and salad (1 cup mixed greens, 1 cup arugula, diced red peppers, 1 diced roma tomato) with 1 tablespoon Balsamic Vinaigrette
Midafternoon Snack	jicama sticks sprinkled with lime juice
Dinner	Grilled Chicken Breast with Roasted Vegetable Salsa served with Zucchini Medley and 1 teaspoon ground flaxseeds
Dessert	½ cup berries

Day 25

Breakfast	Berry Smoothie
Midmorning Snack	apple with 12 almonds
Lunch	3 ounces sliced grilled beef, ¾ cup artichokes mixed with 1 tablespoon vinaigrette, ½ cup cooked barley, Broccolini, and 2 teaspoons ground flaxseeds
Midafternoon Snack	Jicama Sticks with Roasted Red Pepper-White Bean Dip
Dinner	Portobello Mushroom with Chicken Cacciatore and Sautéed Swiss Chard, 1 teaspoon ground flaxseeds, and ½ cup brown rice

Day 26

Breakfast	2 soft-boiled eggs, 2 turkey breakfast links, tomato slices, and 1 slice bread (e.g., rye)
Midmorning Snack	1 cup berries topped with 1 tablespoon sliced almonds
Lunch	Barley-Lentil Soup with Swiss Chard, Chopped Salad, and 1 teaspoon ground flaxseeds
Midafternoon Snack	¾ cup berries with 2 teaspoons toasted ground flaxseeds
Dinner	Thai Coconut Tempeh, ½ cup Roasted Cauliflower Florets, 1 tablespoon ground flaxseeds, and ½ cup cooked brown rice

Day 27

Breakfast	Pumpkin Pie Oatmeal
Midmorning Snack	pear with 12 almonds and Cleansing Lemon Tea
Lunch	Jerusalem Artichoke and Leek Soup, 3 ounces grilled beef or chicken, Arugula Salad with ¾ cup beets, 7 black olives, 1 tablespoon lemon-olive oil vinaigrette topped with 1 ounce feta or low-fat goat cheese, and 1 teaspoon ground flaxseeds
Midafternoon Snack	2 tablespoons Chickpea Dip with pita wedges (a 6½-inch diameter pita) or Flaxseed Crackers
Dinner	Lamb Curry, steamed broccoli, 2 teaspoons ground flaxseeds, and ½ cup cooked brown rice

Day 28

Breakfast	Berry Smoothie
Midmorning Snack	1 slice rye bread with tomato slices drizzled with ½ teaspoon olive oil and balsamic vinegar
Lunch	4 ounces sliced Grilled Chicken Breast, ¾ cup artichokes with 1 tablespoon vinaigrette, Broccolini, 2 teaspoons ground flaxseeds, and Cleansing Lemon Tea
Dinner	Chicken Stir-Fry over "Rice," 1 cup steamed spinach or green beans, 1 teaspoon ground flaxseeds, and ½ cup cooked brown rice or quinoa
Dessert	Microwave Apple Crumble

Resources

The Inside Out Diet
www.iodiet.com
The official site of the Inside Out Diet. You'll find articles, support community, updates, recipes, forums, resources, newsletters, and more to help you in your effort to lose weight and be healthy.

Alternative Medicine site at About.com
www.altmedicine.about.com
This is my alternative medicine Web site at About.com, part of the New York Times Company, where you'll find feature articles, up-to-date links to the best alternative medicine resources on the Web, my popular weekly newsletter, and other health information.

Natural Foods

Yogurt and Kefir

Helios Nutrition (organic kefir with FOS): (888)-3-HELIOS, www.heliosnutrition.com
Horizon Organic: (888) 494-3020 or (303) 443-3470, www.horizonorganic.com
Organic Valley: (888) 444-6455, www.organicvalley.coop
Stonyfield Farm: (800) 776-2697, www.stonyfield.com

Goat Cheese

Fresh Direct: Web site that offers a variety of organic fruit, vegetables, dairy, meat, poultry, and grocery items. Based in Long Island City, New York, the company carries Coach Farm low-fat goat cheese stick.
www.FreshDirect.com

Flax Crackers

Foods Alive: (260) 488-4497, www.foodsalive.com
Matter of Flax: (928) 445-4474, www.matterofflax.com

Almond Milk, plain

Pacific Foods: Makers of almond milk that can be found in many health food stores. (503) 692-9666, www.pacificfoods.com

Oils

Spectrum Naturals: Makers of organic oils, such as extra-virgin olive oil, almond oil, avocado oil, walnut oil, vinegars, and omega-3 organic mayonnaise. www.spectrum organics.com

Avocado Oil

Olivado: www.olivado.com

Macadamia Nut Oil

Nature's Way: www.naturesway.com
NOW Foods: www.nowfoods.com

Omega Fatty Acids

Nordic Naturals: Carries a variety of omega fatty acids. The company's Pro EFA Fish Oil is a 5:1 combination of omega-3 to omega-6 from fish oil and borage oil, with natural lemon extract.
www.nordicnaturals.com

Sweeteners

Yacon Syrup

Rawganique: Online organic raw foods store.
(877) 729-4367, www.rawganique.com

Stevia

Wisdom Natural Brands: (800) 899-9908, www.sweetleaf.com

Organic Poultry and Beef

Applegate Farms: Organic chicken-apple sausage, organic turkey bacon, and deli meats.
(866) 587-5858, www.applegatefarms.com

Eat Wild: Web site that lists companies that sell grass-fed meat.
(866) 453-8489 or (253) 759-2318, www.eatwild.com

Han's All Natural: Chicken breakfast links and chicken sausages.
www.hansallnatural.com

Wellshire Farms: Turkey bacon, turkey sausages, and kielbasa.
(856) 769-8933, www.wellshirefarms.com

Convenience Foods

Amy's Kitchen: Organic convenience foods found in health food stores and supermarkets. Check the sodium content on labels.
(707) 578-7188, www.amys.com

Moosewood: Organic convenience foods found in health food stores and some supermarkets.
(607) 273-9610, www.moosewoodrestaurant.com

Grains

Bob's Red Mill: Grains, beans, gluten-free, oats, cereals.
(800) 349-2173, www.bobsredmill.com

Heartland's Finest: Pasta made from bean flour.
(888) 658-8909, www.heartlandsfinest.com

Lundberg: Brown rice products, including a blend of brown and wild rice.
(530) 882-4551, www.lundberg.com

Nature's Path: Various hot and cold cereals.
(888) 808-9505, www.naturespath.com

Natural Grocers

Diamond Organics: California-based company provides online, telephone, and catalog ordering of organically grown food and other organic products for direct home delivery in the United States.
(888) 674-2642, www.diamondorganics.com

Green People: Selected list of food co-ops and health food stores.
www.greenpeople.org/healthfood.htm

Trader Joe's: More than two hundred stores in the United States. Lower-priced health foods, gourmet foods, and organic meat, fruit, and vegetables. Try the frozen berries, frozen vegetables, nuts, and organic low-fat yogurt.
www.traderjoes.com

Whole Foods Market: Natural and organic foods supermarket with more than 181 stores in North America and the United Kingdom.
www.wholefoodsmarket.com

Wild Oats: Natural foods supermarket chain in the United States and western Canada.
www.wildoats.com

Fitness

About.com Exercise
Certified personal trainer Paige Waehner's site offers comprehensive, practical information. Includes fitness tools and calculators, exercise demos, a beginner's corner, and plenty of workouts that include cardio, strength training, and flexibility workouts for all fitness levels for abs, total body, upper and lower body, and even some Pilates and yoga moves.
www.exercise.about.com

Complementary and Alternative Medicine Resources

About.com Alternative Medicine
Information about herbs, supplements, diets, remedies, finding a practitioner, and more. Popular weekly newsletter and up-to-date links to the best Web resources.
www.altmedicine.about.com

American College for Advancement in Medicine
www.acam.org

Dr. Andrew Weil
www.drweil.com

Herb Research Foundation
www.herbs.org

Holistic Healing
www.healing.about.com

Lime Media
Healthy living Web site, video, television, radio.
www.lime.com

National Center for Complementary and Alternative Medicine
The federal government's agency for scientific research on complementary and alternative
    medicine (CAM). Contains fact sheets on alternative medicine.
www.nccam.nih.gov

National Library of Medicine's CAM on PubMed
The Web's premier medical research source. Offers a searchable database of complemen-
    tary and alternative medicine abstracts and journal references from major medical
    journals.
www.nccam.nih.gov/camonpubmed

News Target
www.newstarget.com

WebMD
Informative general medical Web site. Includes some alternative information.
www.webmd.com

Health Resources

About.com Hepatitis
www.hepatitis.about.com

About.com IBS and Crohn's Disease
www.ibscrohns.about.com

American Liver Foundation
www.liverfoundation.org

Canadian Liver Foundation
www.liver.ca

Celiac Disease Foundation
www.celiac.org

Thyroid-info.com
www.thyroid-info.com

Herbs and Supplements

ConsumerLab.com
333 Mamaroneck Avenue
White Plains, NY 10605
Phone: (914) 722-9149
www.consumerlab.com
Independent testing of herbs and supplements for consumers and health professionals.
   Paid subscription necessary for full access.

Iherb.com
1435 S. Shamrock Avenue
Monrovia, CA 91016
Phone: (888) 792-0028, (626) 358-5678
www.iherb.com

Diet Web Sites

Diets at IVillage.com
www.diet.ivillage.com

Ediets.com
www.ediets.com

Low-Carb Diets
www.lowcarbdiets.about.com

Low-Fat Cooking
www.lowfatcooking.about.com

Nutrition
Nutrition site at About.com
www.nutrition.about.com

Weight Loss
www.weightloss.about.com

Testing Laboratories and Information

Aeron LifeCycles
1933 Davis Street, Suite 310
San Leandro, CA 94577
Phone: (800) 631-7900
www.aeron.com

AquaMD.com
499 Derby Avenue
West Haven, CT 06516

Phone: (866) 278-2634
www.aquamd.com
Private water testing service.

Genova Diagnostics/Great Smokies Diagnostic Laboratory
63 Zillicoa Street
Asheville, NC 28801
Phone: (828) 253-0621
www.gdx.net
Private lab offers the liver detoxification test that can measure and assess specific aspects
   of detoxification.

MetaMetrix
4855 Peachtree Industrial Blvd., Suite 201
Norcross, GA 30092
Phone: (800) 221-4640, (770) 446-5483
www.metametrix.com

Magazines and Newsletters

About Alternative Medicine
www.altmedicine.about.com

Body + Soul
www.marthastewart.com

Mercola.com
www.mercola.com

Books

Better Basics for the Home: Simple Solutions for Less Toxic Living, Annie Berthold-Bond,
   Three Rivers Press, 1999

Clean House Clean Planet, Karen Logan, Pocket Books, 1997

Dr. Melissa Palmer's Guide to Hepatitis and Liver Disease, Melissa Palmer, Avery, 2004

How to Grow Fresh Air: 50 House Plants That Purify Your Home or Office, B. C. Wolverton, Penguin, 1997

*Living Well with Hypothyroidism: What Your Doctor Doesn't Tell You . . . That You Need to
   Know*, Mary J. Shomon, HarperCollins, 2005

Nurture Nature, Nurture Health: Your Health and the Environment, Mitchell Gaynor,
   M.D., Nurture Nature Press, 2005

Silent Snow: The Slow Poisoning of the Arctic, Marla Cone, Grove Press, 2005

Environment and Health Web Sites

Body Burden
The *Oakland Tribune*'s investigation of our chemical "body burden."
www.insidebayarea.com/bodyburden

Collaborative on Health and Environment
The Collaborative on Health and Environment is a nonpartisan partnership working to fur-
    ther knowledge, action, and cooperation regarding environmental contributors to dis-
    ease and other health problems.
www.healthandenvironment.org

Environmental Working Group
Team of scientists, engineers, policy experts, and lawyers that examines government data,
    legal documents, scientific studies, and laboratory tests to expose health and environ-
    mental threats.
www.ewg.org

National Report on Human Exposure to Environmental Chemicals
Report contains chemical exposure information (measured by chemicals in blood or urine)
    for the U.S. population for 38 of 148 chemicals.
www.cdc.gov/exposurereport

References

1. The Liver Link

Delarue J, Matzinger O, Binnert C, et al. 2003. Fish oil prevents the adrenal activation elicited by mental stress in healthy men. *Diabetes Metab* 29 (3): 289–295.

Epel ES, McEwen B, Seeman T, et al. 2000. Stress and body shape: stress-induced cortisol secretion is consistently greater among women with central fat. *Psychosom Med* 62 (5): 623–632.

Epel ES, Lapidus R, McEwen B, Brownell K. 2001. Stress may add bite to appetite in women: a laboratory study of stress-induced cortisol and eating behavior. *Psychoneuroendocrinology* 26 (1): 37–49.

Fernstrom JD, Wurtman RJ. 1971. Brain serotonin content: increase following ingestion of carbohydrate diet. *Science* 174 (13): 1023–1025.

———. 1997. Brain serotonin content: physiological regulation by plasma neutral amino acids. *Obes Res* 5 (4): 377–380.

Flachs P, Horakova O, Brauner P, et al. 2005. Polyunsaturated fatty acids of marine origin upregulate mitochondrial biogenesis and induce beta-oxidation in white fat. *Diabetologia* 48 (11): 2365–2375.

Gluck ME. 2006. Stress response and binge eating disorder. *Appetite* 46 (1): 26–30.

Mendez-Sanchez N, Gonzalez V, Aguayo P, et al. 2001. Fish oil (n-3) polyunsaturated fatty acids beneficially affect biliary cholesterol nucleation time in obese women losing weight. *J Nutr* 131 (9): 2300–2303.

Moyer AE, Rodin J, Grilo CM, et al. 1994. Stress-induced cortisol response and fat distribution in women. *Obes Res* 2 (3): 255–262.

Nanni G, Scheggi S, Leggio B, et al. 2003. Acquisition of an appetitive behavior prevents development of stress-induced neurochemical modifications in rat nucleus accumbens. *J Neurosci Res* 73 (4): 573–580.

Ruzickova J, Rossmeisl M, Prazak T, et al. 2004. Omega-3 PUFA of marine origin limit diet-induced obesity in mice by reducing cellularity of adipose tissue. *Lipids* 39 (12): 1177–1785.

Sanz Sampelayo MR, Fernandez Navarro JR, Hermoso R, Gil Extremera F, Rodriguez Osorio M. 2006. Thermogenesis associated to the intake of a diet non-supplemented or supplemented with n-3 polyunsaturated fatty acid-rich fat, determined in rats receiving the same quantity of metabolizable energy. *Ann Nutr Metab* 50 (3): 184–192.

Vitaliano PP, Russo J, Scanlan JM, Greeno CG. 1996. Weight changes in caregivers of Alzheimer's care recipients: psychobehavioral predictors. *Psychol Aging* 11 (1): 155–163.

Wang GJ, Volkow ND, Logan J, et al. 2001. Brain dopamine and obesity. *Lancet* 357 (9253): 354–357.

Wang J, Akabayashi A, Dourmashkin J, et al. 1998. Neuropeptide Y in relation to carbohydrate intake, corticosterone and dietary obesity. *Brain Res* 802 (1–2): 75–88.

Yehuda S, Rabinovitz S, Mostofsky DI. 2005. Mixture of essential fatty acids lowers test anxiety. *Nutr Neurosci* 8 (4): 265–267.

2. The Risks and Hazards of Dieting

Adachi T, Yasuda K, Mori C, et al. 2005. Promoting insulin secretion in pancreatic islets by means of bisphenol A and nonylphenol via intracellular estrogen receptors. *Food Chem Toxicol* 43 (5): 713–719.

Alonso-Magdalena P, Morimoto S, Ripoll C, Fuentes E, Nadal A. 2006. The estrogenic effect of bisphenol A disrupts pancreatic beta-cell function in vivo and induces insulin resistance. *Environ Health Perspect* 114 (1): 106–112.

Atanasov AG, Nashev LG, Tam S, Baker ME, Odermatt A. 2005. Organotins disrupt the 11beta-hydroxysteroid dehydrogenase type 2-dependent local inactivation of glucocorticoids. *Environ Health Perspect* 113 (11): 1600–1606.

Atanasov AG, Tam S, Rocken JM, Baker ME, Odermatt A. 2003. Inhibition of 11 beta-hydroxysteroid dehydrogenase type 2 by dithiocarbamates. *Biochem Biophys Res Commun* 308 (2): 257–262.

Bigsby RM, Caperell-Grant A, Madhukar BV. 1997. Xenobiotics released from fat during fasting produce estrogenic effects in ovariectomized mice. *Cancer Res* 57 (5): 865–869.

Baillie-Hamilton PF. 2002. Chemical toxins: a hypothesis to explain the global obesity epidemic. *J Altern Complement Med* 8 (2): 185–192.

Boas M, Feldt-Rasmussen U, Skakkebaek NE, Main KM. 2006. Environmental chemicals and thyroid function. *Eur J Endocrinol* 154 (5): 599–611.

Braune BM, Outridge PM, Fisk AT, et al. 2005. Persistent organic pollutants and mercury in marine biota of the Canadian Arctic: an overview of spatial and temporal trends. *Sci Total Environ* 351–352: 4–56.

Carpenter DO. 2006. Polychlorinated biphenyls (PCBs): routes of exposure and effects on human health. *Rev Environ Health* 21 (1): 1–23.

Charlier C, Desaive C, Plomteux G. 2002. Human exposure to endocrine disrupters: consequences of gastroplasty on plasma concentration of toxic pollutants. *Int J Obes Relat Metab Disord* 26 (11): 1465–1468.

Chevrier J, Dewailly E, Ayotte P, et al. 2000. Body weight loss increases plasma and adipose tissue concentrations of potentially toxic pollutants in obese individuals. *Int J Obes Relat Metab Disord* 24 (10): 1272–1278.

Clegg DJ, Brown LM, Woods SC, Benoit SC. 2006. Gonadal hormones determine sensitivity to central leptin and insulin. *Diabetes* 55 (4): 978–987.

Cotrim HP, De Freitas LA, Freitas C, et al. 2004. Clinical and histopathological features of NASH in workers exposed to chemicals with or without associated metabolic conditions. *Liver Int* 24 (2): 131–135.

Dixon JB, Bhathal PS, Hughes NR, O'Brien PE. 2004. Nonalcoholic fatty liver disease: improvement in liver histological analysis with weight loss. *Hepatology* 39 (6): 1647–1654.

Donnelly KL, Smith CI, Schwarzenberg SJ, et al. 2005. Sources of fatty acids stored in the liver and secreted via lipoproteins in patients with nonalcoholic fatty liver disease. *J Clin Invest* 115: 1343–1351.

Eguchi Y, Eguchi T, Mizuta T, et al. 2006. Visceral fat accumulation and insulin resistance are important factors in nonalcoholic fatty liver disease. *J Gastroenterol* 41 (5): 462–469.

Environmental Defence. 2005. "Toxic Nation: A Report on Pollution in Canadians," *Environmental Defence*, www.environmentaldefence.ca/toxicnation/landing.htm. (Accessed February 17, 2006.)

Everett CJ, Frithsen IL, Diaz VA, et al. 2006. Association of a polychlorinated dibenzo-p-dioxin, a polychlorinated biphenyl, and DDT with diabetes in the 1999–2002 National Health and Nutrition Examination Survey. *Environ Res* Dec 20; [Epub ahead of print].

Fierens S, Mairesse H, Heilier JF. 2003. Dioxin/polychlorinated biphenyl body burden, diabetes and endometriosis: findings in a population-based study in Belgium. *Biomarkers* 8 (6): 529–534.

Fischer D. 2005. "A Body's Burden: Our Chemical Legacy," *Oakland Tribune*, www.insidebayarea.com/bodyburden. (Accessed February 17, 2006.)

Flachs P, Horakova O, Brauner P, et al. 2005. Polyunsaturated fatty acids of marine origin upregulate mitochondrial biogenesis and induce beta-oxidation in white fat. *Diabetologia* 48 (11): 2365–2375.

Gill HK, Wu GY. 2006. Non-alcoholic fatty liver disease and the metabolic syndrome: effects of weight loss and a review of popular diets. Are low carbohydrate diets the answer? *World J Gastroenterol* 12 (3): 345–353.

Grun F, Watanabe H, Zamanian Z, et al. 2006. Endocrine-disrupting organotin compounds are potent inducers of adipogenesis in vertebrates. *Mol Endocrinol* 20 (9): 2141–2155.

Hallgren S, Sinjari T, Hakansson H, Darnerud PO. 2001. Effects of polybrominated diphenyl ethers (PBDEs) and polychlorinated biphenyls (PCBs) on thyroid hormone and vitamin A levels in rats and mice. *Arch Toxicol* 75 (4): 200–208.

Heindel JJ. 2003. Endocrine disruptors and the obesity epidemic. *Toxicol Sci* 76 (2): 247–249.

Hue O, Marcotte J, Berrigan F, et al. 2006. Increased plasma levels of toxic pollutants accompanying weight loss induced by hypocaloric diet or by bariatric surgery. *Obes Surg* 16 (9):1145–1154.

Imbeault P, Chevrier J, Dewailly E, et al. 2001. Increase in plasma pollutant levels in response to weight loss in humans is related to in vitro subcutaneous adipocyte basal lipolysis. *Int J Obes Relat Metab Disord* 25 (11): 1585–1591.

Inadera H, Shimomura A. 2005. Environmental chemical tributyltin augments adipocyte differentiation. *Toxicol Lett* 159 (3): 226–234.

Jaga K, Duvvi H. 2001. Risk reduction for DDT toxicity and carcinogenesis through dietary modification. *J R Soc Health* 121 (2): 107–113.

Jandacek RJ, Anderson N, Liu M, et al. 2005. Effects of yo-yo diet, caloric restriction, and olestra on tissue distribution of hexachlorobenzene. *Am J Physiol Gastrointest Liver Physiol* 288 (2): G292–299.

Johnson-Restrepo B, Kannan K, Rapaport DP, Rodan BD. 2005. Polybrominated diphenyl ethers and polychlorinated biphenyls in human adipose tissue from New York. *Environ Sci Technol* 39 (14): 5177–5182.

Kiewiet RM, Durian MF, Van Leersum M, Hesp FL, Van Vliet AC. 2006. Gallstone formation after weight loss following gastric banding in morbidly obese Dutch patients. *Obes Surg* 16 (5): 592–596.

Kitamura S, Kato T, Iida M, et al. 2005. Anti-thyroid hormonal activity of tetrabromobisphenol A, a flame retardant, and related compounds: affinity to the mammalian thyroid hormone receptor, and effect on tadpole metamorphosis. *Life Sci* 76 (14): 1589–1601.

Lordo RA, Dinh KT, Schwemberger JG. 2004. Semivolatile organic compounds in adipose tissue: estimated averages for the U.S. population and selected subpopulations. *Environ Health Perspect* 112: 854–861.

Mendez-Sanchez N, Gonzalez V, Chavez-Tapia N, Ramos MH, Uribe M. 2004. Weight reduction and ursodeoxycholic acid in subjects with nonalcoholic fatty liver disease. A double-blind, placebo-controlled trial. *Ann Hepatol* 3 (3): 108–112.

Milewicz T, Krzysiek J, Janczak-Saif A, et al. 2005. Age, insulin, SHBG and sex steroids exert secondary influence on plasma leptin level in women. *Endokrynol Pol* 56 (6): 883–890.

Moriyama K, Tagami T, Akamizu T, et al. 2002. Thyroid hormone action is disrupted by bisphenol A as an antagonist. *J Clin Endocrinol Metab* 87 (11): 5185–5190.

Moyers B. 2001. "Trade Secrets: A Moyers Report," Public Affairs Television, www.pbs.org/tradesecrets.

Mullerova D, Kopecky J. 2006. White adipose tissue: storage and effector site for environmental pollutants. *Physiol Res*, www.biomd.cas.cz/pphysiolres/pdf/prepress/1022.pdf, pp. 1–17.

Pelletier C, Despres JP, Tremblay A. 2002. Plasma organochlorine concentrations in endurance athletes and obese individuals. *Med Sci Sports Exer* 34 (12): 1971–1975.

Pelletier C, Doucet E, Imbeault P, Tremblay A. 2002. Associations between weight loss-induced changes in plasma organochlorine concentrations, serum T(3) concentration, and resting metabolic rate. *Toxicol Sci* 67 (1): 46–51.

Pelletier C, Imbeault P, Tremblay A. 2003. Energy balance and pollution by organochlorines and polychlorinated biphenyls. *Obes Rev* 4 (1): 17–24.

Petersen KF, Dufour S, Befroy D, et al. 2005. Reversal of nonalcoholic hepatic steatosis, hepatic insulin resistance, and hyperglycemia by moderate weight reduction in patients with type 2 diabetes. *Diabetes* 54 (3): 603–608.

Puder JJ, Monaco SE, Sen Gupta S, et al. 2006. Estrogen and exercise may be related to body fat distribution and leptin in young women. *Fertil Steril* 86 (3): 694–699.

Robinson PE, Mack GA, Remmers J, Levy R, Mohadjer L. 1990. Trends of PCB, hexachlorobenzene, and beta-benzene hexachloride levels in the adipose tissue of the U.S. population. *Environ Res* 53 (2): 175–192.

Roy D, Palangat M, Chen CW, et al. 1997. Biochemical and molecular changes at the cellular level in response to exposure to environmental estrogen-like chemicals. *J Toxicol Environ Health* 50 (1):1–29.

Rylander L, Rignell-Hydbom A, Hagmar L. 2005. A cross-sectional study of the association between persistent organochlorine pollutants and diabetes. *Environ Health* 4:28.

Schnare DW, Denk G, Shields M, Brunton S. 1982. Evaluation of a detoxification regimen for fat stored xenobiotics. *Med Hypotheses* 9 (3): 265–282.

Steinmetz R, Young PC, Caperell-Grant A, et al. 1996. Novel estrogenic action of the pesticide residue beta-hexachlorocyclohexane in human breast cancer cells. *Cancer Res* 56 (23): 5403–409.

Stratopoulos C, Papakonstantinou A, Terzis I, et al. 2005. Changes in liver histology accompanying massive weight loss after gastroplasty for morbid obesity. *Obes Surg* 15 (8): 1154–1160.

Suzuki A, Lindor K, St Saver J, et al. 2005. Effect of changes on body weight and lifestyle in nonalcoholic fatty liver disease. *J Hepatol* 43 (6):1060–1066.

Tremblay A. 2004. Dietary fat and body weight set point. *Nutr Rev* 62 (7 Pt 2): S75–77.

Tremblay A, Pelletier C, Doucet E, Imbeault P. 2004. Thermogenesis and weight loss in obese individuals: a primary association with organochlorine pollution. *Int J Obes Relat Metab Disord* 28 (7): 936–939.

Tsukino H, Hanaoka T, Sasaki H, et al. 2006. Fish intake and serum levels of organochlo-rines among Japanese women. *Sci Total Environ* 359 (1–3): 90–100.

Valtuena S, Pellegrini N, Ardigo D, et al. 2006. Dietary glycemic index and liver steato-sis. *Am J Clin Nutr* 84 (1): 136–142.

Van Oostdam J, Donaldson SG, Feeley M, et al. 2005. Human health implications of envi-ronmental contaminants in Arctic Canada: a review. *Sci Total Environ* 351–352: 165–246.

Vasiliu O, Cameron L, Gardiner J. 2006. Polybrominated biphenyls, polychlorinated biphenyls, body weight, and incidence of adult-onset diabetes mellitus. *Epidemiology* 17 (4): 350–351.

Wanless IR, Lentz JS. 1990. Fatty liver hepatitis (steatohepatitis) and obesity: an autopsy study with analysis of risk factors. *Hepatology* 12 (5): 1106–1110.

Wilson GL, LeDoux SP. 1989. The role of chemicals in the etiology of diabetes mellitus. *Toxicol Pathol* 17 (2): 357–363.

Zhou T, Ross DG, DeVito MJ, Crofton KM. 2001. Effects of short-term in vivo exposure to polybrominated diphenyl ethers on thyroid hormones and hepatic enzyme activities in weanling rats. *Toxicol Sci* 61 (1): 76–82.

Zhou T, Taylor MM, DeVito MJ, Crofton KM. 2002. Developmental exposure to bromi-nated diphenyl ethers results in thyroid hormone disruption. *Toxicol Sci* 66 (1): 105–116.

3. Give Your Tired Liver a Boost

Agarwal M, Srivastava VK, Saxena KK, Kumar A. 2006. Hepatoprotective activity of Beta vulgaris against CCl4-induced hepatic injury in rats. *Fitoterapia* 77 (2): 91–93.

Ahuja KD, Robertson IK, Geraghty DP, Ball MJ. 2006. Effects of chili consumption on postprandial glucose, insulin, and energy metabolism. *Am J Clin Nutr* 84 (1): 63–69.

Andorfer JH, Tchaikovskaya T, Listowsky I. 2004. Selective expression of glutathione S-transferase genes in the murine gastrointestinal tract in response to dietary organo-sulfur compounds. *Carcinogenesis* 25 (3): 359–367.

Asai A, Miyazawa T. 2001. Dietary curcuminoids prevent high-fat diet-induced lipid accu-mulation in rat liver and epididymal adipose tissue. *J Nutr* 131 (11): 2932–2935.

Auer W, Eiber A, Hertkorn E, et al. 1990. Hypertension and hyperlipidaemia: garlic helps in mild cases. *Br J Clin Pract* (Suppl 69): 3–6.

Cankurtaran M, Kav T, Yavuz B, et al. 2006. Serum vitamin-E levels and its relation to clin-ical features in nonalcoholic fatty liver disease with elevated ALT levels. *Acta Gastroen-terol Belg* 69 (1): 5–11.

Carlson DL, Hites RA. 2005. Polychlorinated biphenyls in salmon and salmon feed: global differences and bioaccumulation. *Environ Sci Technol* 39 (19): 7389–7395.

Durak I, Kavutcu M, Aytac B, et al. 2004. Effects of garlic extract consumption on blood lipid and oxidant/antioxidant parameters in humans with high blood cholesterol. *J Nutr Biochem* 15 (6): 373–377.

Foran JA, Carpenter DO, Hamilton MC, Knuth BA, Schwager SJ. 2005. Risk-based con-sumption advice for farmed Atlantic and wild Pacific salmon contaminated with diox-ins and dioxin-like compounds. *Environ Health Perspect* 113 (5): 552–556.

Foran JA, Good DH, Carpenter DO, et al. 2005. Quantitative analysis of the benefits and risks of consuming farmed and wild salmon. *J Nutr* 135 (11): 2639–2643.

Gonen A, Harats D, Rabinkov A, et al. 2005. The antiatherogenic effect of allicin: possi-ble mode of action. *Pathobiology* 72 (6): 325–334.

Gross-Steinmeyer K, Stapleton PL, Liu F, et al. 2004. Phytochemical-induced changes in gene expression of carcinogen-metabolizing enzymes in cultured human primary hepatocytes. *Xenobiotica* 34 (7): 619–632.

Huang X, Hites RA, Foran JA, et al. 2005. Consumption advisories for salmon based on risk of cancer and noncancer health effects. *Environ Res* 101 (2): 263–274.

Iqbal M, Sharma SD, Okazaki Y, Fujisawa M, Okada S. 2003. Dietary supplementation of curcumin enhances antioxidant and phase II metabolizing enzymes in ddY male mice: possible role in protection against chemical carcinogenesis and toxicity. *Pharmacol Toxicol* 92 (1): 33–38.

Ishii Y, Ishida T, Mutoh J, Yamada H, Oguri K. 2005. Possible candidates for the compound which is expected to attenuate dioxin toxicity. *Fukuoka Igaku Zasshi* 96 (5): 204–213.

Katz DL, Evans MA, Nawaz H, et al. 2005. Egg consumption and endothelial function: a randomized controlled crossover trial. *Int J Cardiol* 99 (1): 65–70.

Kensler TW, Chen JG, Egner PA, et al. 2005. Effects of glucosinolate-rich broccoli sprouts on urinary levels of aflatoxin-DNA adducts and phenanthrene tetraols in a randomized clinical trial in He Zuo township, Qidong, People's Republic of China. *Cancer Epidemiol Biomarkers Prev* 14 (11 Pt 1): 2605–2613.

Larrosa M, Gonzalez-Sarrias A, Garcia-Conesa MT, Tomas-Barberan FA, Espin JC. 2006. Urolithins, ellagic acid-derived metabolites produced by human colonic microflora, exhibit estrogenic and antiestrogenic activities. *J Agric Food Chem* 54 (5): 1611–1620.

Lemar KM, Turner MP, Lloyd D. 2002. Garlic (Allium sativum) as an anti-Candida agent: a comparison of the efficacy of fresh garlic and freeze-dried extracts. *J Appl Microbiol* 93 (3): 398–405.

Rahman K, Lowe GM. 2006. Garlic and cardiovascular disease: a critical review. *J Nutr* 136 (3 Suppl): 736S–740S.

Shapiro H, Ashkenazi M, Weizman N, et al. 2006. Curcumin ameliorates acute thioacetamide-induced hepatotoxicity. *J Gastroenterol Hepatol* 21 (2): 358–366.

Shapiro TA, Fahey JW, Dinkova-Kostova AT, et al. 2006. Safety, tolerance, and metabolism of broccoli sprout glucosinolates and isothiocyanates: a clinical phase I study. *Nutr Cancer* 55 (1): 53–62.

Shapiro TA, Fahey JW, Wade KL, Stephenson KK, Talalay P. 2001. Chemoprotective glucosinolates and isothiocyanates of broccoli sprouts: metabolism and excretion in humans. *Cancer Epidemiol Biomarkers Prev* 10 (5): 501–508.

Smedsrod B, Melkko J, Araki N, Sano H, Horiuchi S. 1997. Advanced glycation end products are eliminated by scavenger-receptor-mediated endocytosis in hepatic sinusoidal Kupffer and endothelial cells. *Biochem J* 322 (Pt 2): 567–573.

Song EK, Cho H, Kim JS, et al. 2001. Diarylheptanoids with free radical scavenging and hepatoprotective activity in vitro from Curcuma longa. *Planta Med* 67 (9): 876–877.

Vander Wal JS, Marth JM, Khosla P, Jen KL, Dhurandhar NV. 2005. Short-term effect of eggs on satiety in overweight and obese subjects. *J Am Coll Nutr* 24 (6): 510–515.

Yago MD, Gonzalez V, Serrano P, et al. 2005. Effect of the type of dietary fat on biliary lipid composition and bile lithogenicity in humans with cholesterol gallstone disease. *Nutrition* 21 (3): 339–347.

4. Cleanse Your Colon

Aller R, de Luis DA, Izaola O, et al. 2004. Effect of soluble fiber intake in lipid and glucose levels in healthy subjects: a randomized clinical trial. *Diabetes Res Clin Pract* 65 (1): 7–11.

Bhathena SJ, Ali AA, Haudenschild C, et al. 2003. Dietary flaxseed meal is more protective than soy protein concentrate against hypertriglyceridemia and steatosis of the liver in an animal model of obesity. *J Am Coll Nutr* 22 (2): 157–164.

Birketvedt GS, Aaseth J, Florholmen JR, Ryttig K. 2000. Long-term effect of fibre supplement and reduced energy intake on body weight and blood lipids in overweight subjects. *Acta Medica (Hradec Kralove)* 43 (4): 129–132.

Birketvedt GS, Shimshi M, Erling T, Florholmen J. 2005. Experiences with three different fiber supplements in weight reduction. *Med Sci Monit* 11 (1): PI5–PI8.

Bizeau ME, Pagliassotti MJ. 2005. Hepatic adaptations to sucrose and fructose. *Metabolism* 54 (9): 1189–1201.

Cairella M, Marchini G. 1995. Evaluation of the action of glucomannan on metabolic parameters and on the sensation of satiation in overweight and obese patients. *Clin Ter* 146 (4): 269–274.

Chen J, He J, Wildman RP, et al. 2006. A randomized controlled trial of dietary fiber intake on serum lipids. *Eur J Clin Nutr* 60 (1): 62–68.

Chen HL, Sheu WH, Tai TS, Liaw YP, Chen YC. 2003. Konjac supplement alleviated hypercholesterolemia and hyperglycemia in type 2 diabetic subjects—a randomized double-blind trial. *J Am Coll Nutr* 22 (1): 36–42.

Cunnane SC, Hamadeh MJ, Liede AC, et al. 1995. Nutritional attributes of traditional flaxseed in healthy young adults. *Am J Clin Nutr* 61 (1): 62–68.

Dahl WJ, Lockert EA, Cammer AL, Whiting SJ. 2005. Effects of flax fiber on laxation and glycemic response in healthy volunteers. *J Med Food* 8 (4): 508–511.

Delargy HJ, O'Sullivan KR, Fletcher RJ, Blundell JE. 1997. Effects of amount and type of dietary fibre (soluble and insoluble) on short-term control of appetite. *Int J Food Sci Nutr* 48 (1): 67–77.

Delzenne NM, Cani PD, Daubioul C, Neyrinck AM. 2005. Impact of inulin and oligofructose on gastrointestinal peptides. *Br J Nutr* 93 (Suppl 1): S157–S161.

Endoh D, Okui T, Ozawa S, et al. 2002. Protective effect of a lignan-containing flaxseed extract against CCl(4)-induced hepatic injury. *J Vet Med Sci* 64 (9): 761–765.

Galisteo M, Suarez A, del Pilar Montilla M, et al. 2000. Antihepatotoxic activity of Rosmarinus tomentosus in a model of acute hepatic damage induced by thioacetamide. *Phytother Res* 14 (7): 522–526.

Gruendel S, Garcia AL, Otto B, et al. 2006. Carob pulp preparation rich in insoluble dietary fiber and polyphenols enhances lipid oxidation and lowers postprandial acylated ghrelin in humans. *J Nutr* 136 (6):1533–1538.

Gustafsson U, Wang FH, Axelson M, et al. 1997. The effect of vitamin C in high doses on plasma and biliary lipid composition in patients with cholesterol gallstones: prolongation of the nucleation time. *Eur J Clin Invest* 27 (5): 387–391.

He J, Streiffer RH, Muntner P, Krousel-Wood MA, Whelton PK. 2004. Effect of dietary fiber intake on blood pressure: a randomized, double-blind, placebo-controlled trial. *J Hypertens* 22 (1): 73–80.

Hemmings SJ, Song X. 2005. The effects of dietary flaxseed on the Fischer 344 rat. III. Protection against CCl(4)-induced liver injury. *Cell Biochem Funct* 23 (6): 389–398.

Jenkins DJ, Kendall CW, Vuksan V, et al. 2002. Soluble fiber intake at a dose approved by the U.S. Food and Drug Administration for a claim of health benefits: serum lipid risk factors for cardiovascular disease assessed in a randomized controlled crossover trial. *Am J Clin Nutr* 75 (5): 834–839.

Kang MJ, Kim JI, Yoon SY, Kim JC, Cha IJ. 2006. Pinitol from soybeans reduces postprandial blood glucose in patients with type 2 diabetes mellitus. *J Med Food* 9 (2): 182–186.

Karmally W, Montez MG, Palmas W, et al. 2005. Cholesterol-lowering benefits of oat-containing cereal in Hispanic Americans. *J Am Diet Assoc* 105 (6): 967–970.

Keithley J, Swanson B. 2005. Glucomannan and obesity: a critical review. *Altern Ther Health Med* 11 (6): 30–34.

Kim JI, Kim JC, Kang MJ, et al. 2005. Effects of pinitol isolated from soybeans on glycaemic control and cardiovascular risk factors in Korean patients with type II diabetes mellitus: a randomized controlled study. *Eur J Clin Nutr* 59 (3): 456–458.

Kraft, K. 1997. Artichoke leaf extract-recent findings reflecting effects on lipid metabolism, liver and gastrointestinal tracts. *Phytomedicine* 4:369–378.

Livieri C, Novazi F, Lorini R. 1992. The use of highly purified glucomannan-based fibers in childhood obesity. *Pediatr Med Chir* 14 (2): 195–198.

Moreyra AE, Wilson AC, Koraym A. 2005. Effect of combining psyllium fiber with simvastatin in lowering cholesterol. *Arch Intern Med* 165 (10): 1161–1166.

Owen RW, Haubner R, Hull WE, et al. 2003. Isolation and structure elucidation of the major individual polyphenols in carob fibre. *Food Chem Toxicol* 41 (12): 1727–1738.

Stuglin C, Prasad K. 2005. Effect of flaxseed consumption on blood pressure, serum lipids, hemopoietic system and liver and kidney enzymes in healthy humans. *J Cardiovasc Pharmacol Ther* 10 (1): 23–27.

Vita PM, Restelli A, Caspani P, Klinger R. 1992. Chronic use of glucomannan in the dietary treatment of severe obesity. *Minerva Med* 83 (3): 135–139.

Walsh DE, Yaghoubian V, Behforooz A. 1984. Effect of glucomannan on obese patients: a clinical study. *Int J Obes* 8 (4): 289–293.

Wang L, Chen J, Thompson LU. 2005. The inhibitory effect of flaxseed on the growth and metastasis of estrogen receptor negative human breast cancer xenograftsis attributed to both its lignan and oil components. *Int J Cancer* 116 (5): 793–798.

Zunft HJ, Luder W, Harde A, et al. 2003. Carob pulp preparation rich in insoluble fibre lowers total and LDL cholesterol in hypercholesterolemic patients. *Eur J Nutr* 42 (5): 235–242.

5. Restore Insulin and Leptin Sensitivity to Burn Fat

Aguilera CM, Ramirez-Tortosa CL, Quiles JL, et al. 2005. Monounsaturated and omega-3 but not omega-6 polyunsaturated fatty acids improve hepatic fibrosis in hypercholesterolemic rabbits. *Nutrition* 21 (3): 363–371.

Bantle JP. 2006. Is fructose the optimal low glycemic index sweetener? *Nestle Nutr Workshop Ser Clin Perform Programme* 11: 83–95.

Berard AM, Dumon MF, Darmon M. 2004. Dietary fish oil up-regulates cholesterol 7 alpha-hydroxylase mRNA in mouse liver leading to an increase in bile acid and cholesterol excretion. *FEBS Lett* 559 (1–3): 125–128.

Carpentier YA, Portois L, Malaisse WJ. 2006. N-3 fatty acids and the metabolic syndrome. *Am J Clin Nutr* 83 (6 Suppl): 1499S–1504S.

Costarelli V, Sanders TA. 2001. Acute effects of dietary fat composition on postprandial plasma bile acid and cholecystokinin concentrations in healthy premenopausal women. *Br J Nutr* 86 (4): 471–477.

Faeh D, Minehira K, Schwarz JM, et al. 2005. Effect of fructose overfeeding and fish oil administration on hepatic de novo lipogenesis and insulin sensitivity in healthy men. *Diabetes* 54 (7): 1907–1913.

Fraquelli M, Pagliarulo M, Colucci A, Paggi S, Conte D. 2003. Gallbladder motility in obesity, diabetes mellitus and coeliac disease. *Dig Liver Dis* 35 (Suppl 3): S12–16.

Gaby AR. 2005. Adverse effects of dietary fructose. *Altern Med Rev* 10 (4): 294–306.

Gregersen S, Jeppesen PB, Holst JJ, Hermansen K. 2004. Antihyperglycemic effects of stevioside in type 2 diabetic subjects. *Metabolism* 53 (1): 73–76.

Grimsgaard S, Bonaa KH, Hansen JB, et al. 1997. Highly purified eicosapentaenoic acid and docosahexaenoic acid in humans have similar triacylglycerol-lowering effects but divergent effects on serum fatty acids. *Am J Clin Nutr* 66 (3): 649–659.

Harris WS. 1997. N-3 fatty acids and serum lipoproteins: human studies. *Am J Clin Nutr* 65 (5 Suppl): 1645S–1654S.

Harris WS, Dujovne CA, Zucker M, et al. 1988. Effects of a low saturated fat, low cholesterol fish oil supplement in hypertriglyceridemic patients. A placebo-controlled trial. *Ann Intern Med* 109 (6): 465–470.

Houten SM, Watanabe M, Auwerx J. 2006. Endocrine functions of bile acids. *EMBO J* 25 (7): 1419–1425.

Jonkers IJ, Smelt AH, Princen HM, et al. 2006. Fish oil increases bile acid synthesis in male patients with hypertriglyceridemia. *J Nutr* 136 (4): 987–991.

Khan A, Safdar M, Ali Khan MM, et al. 2003. Cinnamon improves glucose and lipids of people with type 2 diabetes. *Diabetes Care* 26 (12): 3215–3218.

Kim SH, Hyun SH, Choung SY. 2006. Anti-diabetic effect of cinnamon extract on blood glucose in db/db mice. *J Ethnopharmacol* 104 (1–2): 119–123.

Kusano S, Abe H, Tamura H. 2001. Isolation of antidiabetic components from white-skinned sweet potato (Ipomoea batatas L.). *Biosci Biotechnol Biochem* 65 (1): 109–114.

Lands WEM, Libelt B, Morris A, et al. 1992. Maintenance of lower proportions of n-6 eicosanoid precursors in phospholipids of human plasma in response to added dietary n-3 fatty acids. *Biochem Biophys Acta* 180: 147–162.

Ludvik B, Waldhausl W, Prager R, Kautzky-Willer A, Pacini G. 2003. Mode of action of ipomoea batatas (Caiapo) in type 2 diabetic patients. *Metabolism* 52 (7): 875–880.

Mang B, Wolters M, Schmitt B, et al. 2006. Effects of a cinnamon extract on plasma glucose, HbA, and serum lipids in diabetes mellitus type 2. *Eur J Clin Invest* 36 (5): 340–344.

Matsui T, Ebuchi S, Kobayashi M, et al. 2002. Anti-hyperglycemic effect of diacylated anthocyanin derived from Ipomoea batatas cultivar Ayamurasaki can be achieved through the alpha-glucosidase inhibitory action. *J Agric Food Chem* 50 (25): 7244–7248.

Montori VM, Farmer A, Wollan PC, et al. 2000. Fish oil supplementation in type 2 diabetes: a quantitative systematic review. *Diabetes Care* 23 (9): 1407–1415.

Nordoy A, Bonaa KH, Sandset PM, et al. 2000. Effect of omega-3 fatty acids and simvastatin on hemostatic risk factors and postprandial hyperlipemia in patients with combined hyperlipemia. *Arterioscler Thromb Vasc Biol* 20 (1): 259–265.

Pereira MA, Swain J, Goldfine AB, et al. 2004. Effects of a low-glycemic load diet on resting energy expenditure and heart disease risk factors during weight loss. *JAMA* 292 (20): 2482–2490.

Roche HM, Gibney MJ. 1996. Postprandial triacylglycerolaemia: the effect of low-fat dietary treatment with and without fish oil supplementation. *Eur J Clin Nutr* 50 (9): 617–624.

Rodriguez-Hernandez H, Gonzalez JL, Rodriguez-Moran M, et al. 2005. Hypomagnesemia, insulin resistance, and non-alcoholic steatohepatitis in obese subjects. *Arch Med Res* 36 (4): 362–366.

Sanders TA, Oakley FR, Miller GJ, et al. 1997. Influence of n-6 versus n-3 polyunsaturated fatty acids in diets low in saturated fatty acids on plasma lipoproteins and hemostatic factors. *Arterioscler Thromb Vasc Biol* 17 (12): 3449–3460.

Sera N, Morita K, Nagasoe M, et al. 2005. Binding effect of polychlorinated compounds and environmental carcinogens on rice bran fiber. *J Nutr Biochem* 16 (1): 50–58.

Suzuki YA, Murata Y, Inui H, Sugiura M, Nakano Y. 2005. Triterpene glycosides of Siraitia grosvenori inhibit rat intestinal maltase and suppress the rise in blood glucose level after a single oral administration of maltose in rats. *J Agric Food Chem* 53 (8): 2941–2946.

Taher M, Abdul Majid FA, Sarmidi MR. 2004. Cinnamtannin B1 activity on adipocytes formation. *Med J Malaysia* 59 (Suppl B): 97–98.

Takeo E, Yoshida H, Tada N, et al. 2002. Sweet elements of Siraitia grosvenori inhibit oxidative modification of low-density lipoprotein. *J Atheroscler Thromb* 9 (2): 114–120.

Teff KL, Elliott SS, Tschop M, et al. 2004. Dietary fructose reduces circulating insulin and leptin, attenuates postprandial suppression of ghrelin, and increases triglycerides in women. *J Clin Endocrinol Metab* 89 (6): 2963–2972.

Tsai CJ, Leitzmann MF, Willett WC, Giovannucci EL. 2005. Dietary carbohydrates and glycaemic load and the incidence of symptomatic gall stone disease in men. *Gut* 54 (6): 823–828.

Valtuena S, Pellegrini N, Ardigo D, et al. 2006. Dietary glycemic index and liver steatosis. *Am J Clin Nutr* 84 (1): 136–142.

Verspohl EJ, Bauer K, Neddermann E. 2005. Antidiabetic effect of Cinnamomum cassia and Cinnamomum zeylanicum in vivo and in vitro. *Phytother Res* 19 (3): 203–206.

Watanabe M, Houten SM, Mataki C, et al. 2006. Bile acids induce energy expenditure by promoting intracellular thyroid hormone activation. *Nature* 439 (7075): 484–489.

6. Check for Food Intolerances

Breneman JC. 1978. *Basics of Food Allergy*. Springfield, IL: Charles C. Thomas.

Dickey L (ed.). 1976. *Clinical Ecology*. Springfield, IL: Charles C. Thomas.

Drago S, El Asmar R, Di Pierro M, et al. 2006. Gliadin, zonulin and gut permeability: effects on celiac and non-celiac intestinal mucosa and intestinal cell lines. *Scand J Gastroenterol* 41 (4): 408–419.

Freeman HJ. 2006. Hepatobiliary and pancreatic disorders in celiac disease. *World J Gastroenterol* 12 (10): 1503–1508.

Kaukinen K, Halme L, Collin P, et al. 2002. Celiac disease in patients with severe liver disease: gluten-free diet may reverse hepatic failure. *Gastroenterology* 122 (4): 881–888.

Ledochowski M, Widner B, Murr C, Sperner-Unterwger B, Fuchs D. 2001. Fructose malabsorption is associated with decreased plasma tryptophan. *Scand J Gastroenterology* 36 (4): 367–371.

Leffler DA, Kelly CP. 2006. Update on the evaluation and diagnosis of celiac disease. *Curr Opin Allergy Clin Immunol* 6 (3): 191–196.

Meisel H, Fitzgerald RJ. 2000. Opioid peptides encrypted in intact milk protein sequences. *Br J Nutrition* 84 (Suppl 1): S27–31.

Oso O, Fraser NC. 2006. A boy with coeliac disease and obesity. *Acta Paediatr* 95 (5): 618–619.

Page SR, Lloyd CA, Hill PG, Peacock I, Holmes GK. 1994. The prevalence of coeliac disease in adult diabetes mellitus. *QJM* 87 (10): 631–637.

Pimentel M, Chow EJ, Lin HC. 2000. Eradication of small intestinal bacterial overgrowth reduces symptoms of irritable bowel syndrome. *Am J Gastroenterol* 95: 3503–3506.

Rampertab SD, Pooran N, Brar P, Singh P, Green PH. 2006. Trends in the presentation of celiac disease. *Am J Med* 119 (4): 355.e9–14.

Schams D, Karg H. Hormones in milk. 1986. *Ann NY Acad Sci* 464: 75–86.

Teschemacher H, Koch G. 1991. Opioids in milk. *Endocr Regul* 25 (3): 147–150.

Teschemacher H, Koch G, Brantl V. 1997. Milk protein-derived opioid receptor ligands. *Biopolymers* 43 (2): 99–117.

Trompette A, Claustre J, Caillon F, et al. 2003. Milk bioactive peptides and beta-casomorphins induce mucus release in rat jejunum. *J Nutr* 133 (11): 3499–3503.

Zarkadas M, Cranney A, Case S, et al. 2006. The impact of a gluten-free diet on adults with coeliac disease: results of a national survey. *J Hum Nutr Diet* 19 (1): 41–49.

7. Nourish Your Body to Tame Stress Fat

Berube-Parent S, Pelletier C, Dore J, Tremblay A. 2005. Effects of encapsulated green tea and Guarana extracts containing a mixture of epigallocatechin-3-gallate and caffeine on 24 h energy expenditure and fat oxidation in men. *Br J Nutr* 94 (3): 432–436.

Center for Science in the Public Interest. 1996. "The Caffeine Corner: Products Ranked by Amount," *Nutrition Action Health Letter*, www.cspinet.org/nah/caffeine/caffeine_corner.htm. (Accessed March 23, 2006.)

Diepvens K, Kovacs EM, Nijs IM, et al. 2005. Effect of green tea on resting energy expenditure and substrate oxidation during weight loss in overweight females. *Br J Nutr* 94 (6): 1026–1034.

Dudka J, Jodynis-Liebert J, Korobowicz E, et al. 2005. Activity of NADPH-cytochrome P-450 reductase of the human heart, liver and lungs in the presence of (-)-epigallocatechin gallate, quercetin and resveratrol: an in vitro study. *Basic Clin Pharmacol Toxicol* 97 (2): 74–79.

Dulloo AG, Duret C, Rohrer D, et al. 1999. Efficacy of a green tea extract rich in catechin polyphenols and caffeine in increasing 24-h energy expenditure and fat oxidation in humans. *Am J Clin Nutr* 70 (6): 1040–1045.

El-Beshbishy HA. 2005. Protective effect of green tea (Camellia sinensis) extract against tamoxifen-induced liver injury in rats. *J Biochem Mol Biol* 38 (5): 563–570.

Eybl V, Kotyzova D, Koutensky J. 2006. Comparative study of natural antioxidants—curcumin, resveratrol and melatonin—in cadmium-induced oxidative damage in mice. *Toxicology* 225 (2–3): 150–156.

Fiorini RN, Donovan JL, Rodwell D, et al. 2005. Short-term administration of (-)-epigallocatechin gallate reduces hepatic steatosis and protects against warm hepatic ischemia/reperfusion injury in steatotic mice. *Liver Transpl* 11 (3): 298–308.

Hasegawa R, Takeida K, et al. 1998. Inhibitory effect of green tea infusion of hepatotoxicity. *Kokuritsu Iyakuhin Shokuhin Eisei Kenkyusho Hokoku* 116:82–91.

He K, Hu FB, Colditz GA, et al. 2004. Changes in intake of fruits and vegetables in relation to risk of obesity and weight gain among middle-aged women. *Int J Obes Relat Metab Disord* 28 (12): 1569–1574.

Hirano-Ohmori R, Takahashi R, Momiyama Y, et al. 2005. Green tea consumption and serum malondialdehyde-modified LDL concentrations in healthy subjects. *J Am Coll Nutr* 24 (5): 342–346.

Klatsky AL, Morton C, Udaltsova N, Friedman GD. 2006. Coffee, cirrhosis, and transaminase enzymes. *Arch Intern Med* 166 (11): 1190–1195.

Link LB, Potter JD. 2004. Raw versus cooked vegetables and cancer risk. *Cancer Epidemiol Biomarkers Prev* 13 (9): 1422–1435.

Lovallo WR, Whitsett TL, al'Absi M, et al. 2005. Caffeine stimulation of cortisol secretion across waking hours in relation to caffeine intake levels. *Psychosom Med* 67 (5): 734–739.

McKay DL, Blumberg JB. 2007. A review of the bioactivity of South African herbal teas: rooibos (Aspalathus linearis) and honeybush (Cyclopia intermedia). *Phytother Res* 21 (1): 1–16.

Morita K, Matsueda T, Iida T. 1997. Effect of green tea (matcha) on gastrointestinal tract absorption of polychlorinated biphenyls, polychlorinated dibenzofurans and polychlorinated dibenzo-p-dioxins in rats. *Fukuoka Igaku Zasshi* 88 (5): 162–168.

Oak MH, El Bedoui J, Schini-Kerth VB. 2005. Antiangiogenic properties of natural polyphenols from red wine and green tea. *J Nutr Biochem* 16 (1): 1–8.

Ohmori R, Iwamoto T, Tago M, et al. 2005. Antioxidant activity of various teas against free radicals and LDL oxidation. *Lipids* 40 (8): 849–853.

Ozercan IH, Dagli AF, Ustundag B, et al. 2006. Does instant coffee prevent acute liver injury induced by carbon tetrachloride (CCl(4))? *Hepatol Res* 35 (3): 163–168.

Ruhl CE, Everhart JE. 2005. Coffee and tea consumption are associated with a lower incidence of chronic liver disease in the United States. *Gastroenterology* 129 (6): 1928–1936.
———. 2005. Coffee and caffeine consumption reduce the risk of elevated serum alanine aminotransferase activity in the United States. *Gastroenterology* 128 (1): 24–32.

Singal A, Tirkey N, Pilkhwal S, Chopra K. 2006. Green tea (Camellia sinensis) extract ameliorates endotoxin induced sickness behavior and liver damage in rats. *Phytother Res* 20 (2): 125–129.

Sumpio BE, Cordova AC, Berke-Schlessel DW, Qin F, Chen QH. 2006. Green tea, the "Asian paradox," and cardiovascular disease. *J Am Coll Surg* 202 (5): 813–825.

Tian WX. 2006. Inhibition of fatty acid synthase by polyphenols. *Curr Med Chem* 13 (8): 967–977.

Van der Merwe JD, Joubert E, Richards ES, et al. 2006. A comparative study on the antimutagenic properties of aqueous extracts of Aspalathus linearis (rooibos), different Cyclopia spp. (honeybush) and Camellia sinensis teas. *Mutat Res* 611 (1–2): 42–53.

Weiss DJ, Anderton CR. 2003. Determination of catechins in matcha green tea by micellar electrokinetic chromatography. *J Chromatogr A* 1011 (1–2): 173–180.

Westerterp-Plantenga MS, Lejeune MP, Kovacs EM. 2005. Body weight loss and weight maintenance in relation to habitual caffeine intake and green tea supplementation. *Obes Res* 13 (7): 1195–1204.

Wolfram S, Wang Y, Thielecke F. 2006. Anti-obesity effects of green tea: from bedside to bench. *Mol Nutr Food Res* 50 (2): 176–187.

8. Jump-Start Your Detox

Kuligowski J, Halperin KM. 1992. Stainless steel cookware as a significant source of nickel, chromium, and iron. *Arch Environ Contam Toxicol* 23 (2): 211–215.

Powley CR, Michalczyk MJ, Kaiser MA, Buxton LW. 2005. Determination of perfluorooctanoic acid (PFOA) extractable from the surface of commercial cookware under simulated cooking conditions by LC/MS/MS. *Analyst* 130 (9): 1299–1302.

11. Daily Essentials: Exercise, Relaxation, Sleep, Healthy Home, and Journaling

Allison DB, Faith MS. Hypnosis as an adjunct to cognitive-behavioral psychotherapy for obesity: a meta-analytic reappraisal. *J Consult Clin Psychol* 64 (3): 513–516.

Butte W, Heinzow B. 2002. Pollutants in house dust as indicators of indoor contamination. *Rev Environ Contam Toxicol* 175:1–46.

Donnelly JE, Hill JO, Jacobsen DJ, et al. 2003. Effects of a 16-month randomized controlled exercise trial on body weight and composition in young, overweight men and women: the Midwest Exercise Trial. *Arch Intern Med* 163 (11): 1343–1350.

Gangwisch JE, Malaspina D, Boden-Albala B, Heymsfield SB. 2005. Inadequate sleep as a risk factor for obesity: analyses of the NHANES I. *Sleep* 28 (10): 1289–1296.

Godin G, Shepherd RJ. 1985. A simple method to assess exercise behavior in the community. *Can J Appl Sport Sci* 10:141–146.

Hasler G, Buysse DJ, Klaghofer R, et al. 2004. The association between short sleep duration and obesity in young adults: a 13-year prospective study. *Sleep* 27 (4): 661–666.

Jakicic JM, Otto AD. 2006. Treatment and prevention of obesity: what is the role of exercise? *Nutr Rev* 64 (2 Pt 2): S57–61.

Jakicic JM, Marcus BH, Gallagher KI, et al. 2003. Effect of exercise duration and intensity on weight loss in overweight, sedentary women: a randomized trial. *JAMA* 290 (10): 1323–1330.

Jakicic JM, Wing RR, Butler BA, Robertson RJ. 1995. Prescribing exercise in multiple short bouts versus one continuous bout: effects on adherence, cardiorespiratory fitness, and weight loss in overweight women. *Int J Obes Relat Metab Disord* 19 (12): 893–901.

Kirsch I. 1996. Hypnotic enhancement of cognitive-behavioral weight loss treatments—another meta-reanalysis. *J Consult Clin Psychol* 64 (3): 517–519.

Pawlow LA, O'Neil PM, Malcolm RJ. 2003. Night eating syndrome: effects of brief relaxation training on stress, mood, hunger, and eating patterns. *Int J Obes Relat Metab Disord* 27 (8): 970–978.

Perri MG, Anton SD, Durning PE, et al. 2002. Adherence to exercise prescriptions: effects of prescribing moderate versus higher levels of intensity and frequency. *Health Psychol* 21 (5): 452–458.

Rudel RA, Camann DE, Spengler JD, et al. 2003. Phthalates, alkylphenols, pesticides, polybrominated diphenyl ethers, and other endocrine-disrupting compounds in indoor air and dust. *Environ Sci Technol* 37 (20): 4543–4553.

Shaw K, O'Rourke P, Del Mar C, Kenardy J. 2005. Psychological interventions for overweight or obesity. *Cochrane Database Syst Rev* 18 (2): CD003818.

Spiegel K, Knutson K, Leproult R, Tasali E, Van Cauter E. 2005. Sleep loss: a novel risk factor for insulin resistance and type 2 diabetes. *J Appl Physiol* 99 (5): 2008–2019.

Spiegel K, Tasali E, Penev P, Van Cauter E. 2004. Brief communication: Sleep curtailment in healthy young men is associated with decreased leptin levels, elevated ghrelin levels, and increased hunger and appetite. *Ann Intern Med* 141 (11): 846–850.

Stapleton HM, Dodder NG, Offenberg JH, Schantz MM, Wise SA. 2005. Polybrominated diphenyl ethers in house dust and clothes dryer lint. *Environ Sci Technol* 39 (4): 925–931.

Wolverton, B. C. 1997. *How to Grow Fresh Air: 50 House Plants That Purify Your Home or Office.* New York: Penguin Books.

12. Supplements

Abramowicz WN, Galloway SD. 2005. Effects of acute versus chronic L-carnitine L-tartrate supplementation on metabolic responses to steady state exercise in males and females. *Int J Sport Nutr Exerc Metab* 15 (4): 386–400.

Al Faraj S. 2005. Antagonism of the anticoagulant effect of warfarin caused by the use of Commiphora molmol as a herbal medication: a case report. *Ann Trop Med Parasitol* 99 (2): 219–220.

Bach AC, Ingenbleek Y, Frey A. 1996. The usefulness of dietary medium-chain triglycerides in body weight control: fact or fancy? *J Lipid Res* 37:708–726.

Bagchi D, Stohs SJ, Downs BW, Bagchi M, Preuss HG. 2002. Cytotoxicity and oxidative mechanisms of different forms of chromium. *Toxicology* 180 (1): 5–22.

Basch E, Gabardi S, Ulbricht C. 2003. Bitter melon (Momordica charantia): a review of efficacy and safety. *Am J Health Syst Pharm* 60 (4): 356–359.

Baskaran K, Kizar Ahamath B, Radha Shanmugasundaram K, Shanmugasundaram ER. 1990. Antidiabetic effect of a leaf extract from Gymnema sylvestre in non-insulin-dependent diabetes mellitus patients. *J Ethnopharmacol* 30 (3): 295–300.

Bent S, Padula A, Neuhaus J. 2004. Safety and efficacy of citrus aurantium for weight loss. *Am J Cardiol* 94 (10): 1359–1361.

Bianchi A, Cantu P, Firenzuoli F, et al. 2004. Rhabdomyolysis caused by Commiphora mukul, a natural lipid-lowering agent. *Ann Pharmacother* 38 (7–8): 1222–1225.

Broad EM, Maughan RJ, Galloway SD. 2005. Effects of four weeks L-carnitine L-tartrate ingestion on substrate utilization during prolonged exercise. *Int J Sport Nutr Exer Metab* 15 (6): 665–679.

Bruno M, Fiori M, Mattei D, et al. 2006. ELISA and LC-MS/MS methods for determining cyanobacterial toxins in blue-green algae food supplements. *Nat Prod Res* 20 (9): 827–834.

Bui LT, Nguyen DT, Ambrose PJ. 2006. Blood pressure and heart rate effects following a single dose of bitter orange. *Ann Pharmacother* 40 (1): 53–57.

Cangiano C, Ceci F, Cascino A, et al. 1992. Eating behavior and adherence to dietary prescriptions in obese adult subjects treated with 5-hydroxytryptophan. *Am J Clin Nutr* 56 (5): 863–867.

Cangiano C, Laviano A, Del Ben M, et al. 1998. Effects of oral 5-hydroxy-tryptophan on energy intake and macronutrient selection in non-insulin dependent diabetic patients. *Int J Obes Relat Metab Disord* 22 (7): 648–654.

Cater NB, Heller HJ, Denke MA. 1997. Comparison of the effects of medium-chain triacylglycerols, palm oil, and high oleic acid sunflower oil on plasma triacylglycerol fatty acids and lipid and lipoprotein concentrations in humans. *Am J Clin Nutr* 65:41–45.

Ceci F, Cangiano C, Cairella M, et al. 1989. The effects of oral 5-hydroxytryptophan administration on feeding behavior in obese adult female subjects. *J Neural Transm* 76 (2): 109–117.

Colombani P, Wenk C, Kunz I, et al. 1996. Effects of L-carnitine supplementation on physical performance and energy metabolism of endurance-trained athletes: a double-blind crossover field study. *Eur J Appl Physiol Occup Physiol* 73 (5): 434–439.

Crawford V, Scheckenbach R, Preuss HG. 1999. Effects of niacin-bound chromium supplementation on body composition in overweight African-American women. *Diabetes Obes Metab* 1 (6): 331–337.

Gange CA, Madias C, Felix-Getzik EM, et al. 2006. Variant angina associated with bitter orange in a dietary supplement. *Mayo Clin Proc* 81(4): 545–548.

Gilroy DJ, Kauffman KW, Hall RA, Huang X, Chu FS. 2000. Assessing potential health risks from microcystin toxins in blue-green algae dietary supplements. *Environ Health Perspect* 108 (5): 435–439.

Goldenberg D, Golz A, Joachims HZ. 2003. The beverage mate: a risk factor for cancer of the head and neck. *Head Neck* 25 (7): 595–601.

Gunton JE, Cheung NW, Hitchman R, et al. 2005. Chromium supplementation does not improve glucose tolerance, insulin sensitivity, or lipid profile: a randomized, placebo-controlled, double-blind trial of supplementation in subjects with impaired glucose tolerance. *Diabetes Care* 28 (3): 712–713.

Heymsfield SB, Allison DB, Vasselli JR, et al. 1998. Garcinia cambogia (hydroxycitric acid) as a potential antiobesity agent: a randomized controlled trial. *JAMA* 280 (18): 1596–1600.

Hirooka T, Nagase H, Uchida K, et al. 2005. Biodegradation of bisphenol A and disappearance of its estrogenic activity by the green alga Chlorella fusca var. vacuolata. *Environ Toxicol Chem* 24 (8): 1896–1901.

Kleefstra N, Houweling ST, Jansman FG, et al. 2006. Chromium treatment has no effect in patients with poorly controlled, insulin-treated type 2 diabetes in an obese Western population: a randomized, double-blind, placebo-controlled trial. *Diabetes Care* 29 (3): 521–525.

Kovacs EM, Westerterp-Plantenga MS, Saris WH. 2001. The effects of 2-week ingestion of (-)-hydroxycitrate and (-)-hydroxycitrate combined with medium-chain triglycerides on satiety, fat oxidation, energy expenditure and body weight. *Int J Obes Relat Metab Disord* 25 (7): 1087–1094.

Kriketos AD, Thompson HR, Greene H, Hill JO. 1999. (-)-Hydroxycitric acid does not affect energy expenditure and substrate oxidation in adult males in a post-absorptive state. *Int J Obes Relat Metab Disord* 23 (8): 867–873.

Larsen TM, Toubro S, Gudmundsen O, Astrup A. 2006. Conjugated linoleic acid supplementation for 1 y does not prevent weight or body fat regain. *Am J Clin Nutr* 83 (3): 606–612.

Lemon CH, Imoto T, Smith DV. 2003. Differential gurmarin suppression of sweet taste responses in rat solitary nucleus neurons. *J Neurophysiol* 90 (2): 911–923.

Lim K, Ryu S, Nho HS, et al. 2003. (-)-Hydroxycitric acid ingestion increases fat utilization during exercise in untrained women. *J Nutr Sci Vitaminol (Tokyo)* 49 (3): 163–167.

Lima WP, Carnevali LC Jr, Eder R, et al. 2005. Lipid metabolism in trained rats: effect of guarana (Paullinia cupana Mart.) supplementation. *Clin Nutr* 24 (6): 1019–1028.

Livolsi JM, Adams GM, Laguna PL. 2001. The effect of chromium picolinate on muscular strength and body composition in women athletes. *J Strength Cond Res* 15 (2): 161–166.

Luo H, Kashiwagi A, Shibahara T, Yamada K. 2006. Decreased bodyweight without rebound and regulated lipoprotein metabolism by gymnemate in genetic multifactor syndrome animal. *Mol Cell Biochem* May 12, 2006; www.springerlink.metapress.com/content/x063r5wpx2j4q750/fulltext.pdf.

Malewicz B, Wang Z, Jiang C, et al. 2006. Enhancement of mammary carcinogenesis in two rodent models by silymarin dietary supplements. *Carcinogenesis* 27 (9): 1739–1747.

Mattes RD, Bormann L. 2000. Effects of (-)-hydroxycitric acid on appetitive variables. *Physiol Behav* 71 (1–2): 87–94.

Mhurchu CN, Dunshea-Mooij C, Bennett D, Rodgers A. 2005. Effect of chitosan on weight loss in overweight and obese individuals: a systematic review of randomized controlled trials. *Obes Rev* 6 (1): 35–42.

Mhurchu CN, Poppitt SD, McGill AT, et al. 2004. The effect of the dietary supplement, Chitosan, on body weight: a randomised controlled trial in 250 overweight and obese adults. *Int J Obes Relat Metab Disord* 28 (9): 1149–1156.

Min B, McBride BF, Kardas MJ, et al. 2005. Electrocardiographic effects of an ephedra-free, multicomponent weight-loss supplement in healthy volunteers. *Pharmacotherapy* 25 (5): 654–659.

Nadir A, Reddy D, Van Thiel DH. 2000. Cascara sagrada-induced intrahepatic cholestasis causing portal hypertension: case report and review of herbal hepatotoxicity. *Am J Gastroenterol* 95 (12): 3634–3637.

Nakano S, Noguchi T, Takekoshi H, Suzuki G, Nakano M. 2005. Maternal-fetal distribution and transfer of dioxins in pregnant women in Japan, and attempts to reduce maternal transfer with Chlorella (Chlorella pyrenoidosa) supplements. *Chemosphere* 61 (9): 1244–1255.

Ni Mhurchu C, Dunshea-Mooij CA, Bennett D, Rodgers A. 2005. Chitosan for overweight or obesity. *Cochrane Database Syst Rev* 20 (3): CD003892.

Ohia SE, Awe SO, LeDay AM, Opere CA, Bagchi D. 2001. Effect of hydroxycitric acid on serotonin release from isolated rat brain cortex. *Res Commun Mol Pathol Pharmacol* 109 (3–4): 210–216.

Ohkawa S, Yoneda Y, Ohsumi Y, Tabuchi M. 1995. Warfarin therapy and chlorella. *Rinsho Shinkeigaku* 35 (7): 806–807.

Pittler MH. 2003. Chromium picolinate for reducing body weight: meta-analysis of randomized trials. *Int J Obes Relat Metab Disord* 27 (4): 522–529.

Pittler MH, Abbot NC, Harkness EF, Ernst E. 1999. Randomized, double-blind trial of chitosan for body weight reduction. *Eur J Clin Nutr* 53 (5): 379–381.

Poirier H, Shapiro JS, Kim RJ, Lazar MA. 2006. Nutritional supplementation with trans-10, cis-12-conjugated linoleic acid induces inflammation of white adipose tissue. *Diabetes* 55 (6): 1634–1641.

Ramakers JD, Plat J, Sebedio JL, Mensink RP. 2005. Effects of the individual isomers cis-9, trans-11 vs. trans-10, cis-12 of conjugated linoleic acid (CLA) on inflammation parameters in moderately overweight subjects with LDL-phenotype B. *Lipids* 40 (9): 909–918.

Riserus U, Arner P, Brismar K, Vessby B. 2002. Treatment with dietary trans-10, cis-12 conjugated linoleic acid causes isomer-specific insulin resistance in obese men with the metabolic syndrome. *Diabetes Care* 25 (9): 1516–1521.

Riserus U, Basu S, Jovinge S, et al. 2002. Supplementation with conjugated linoleic acid causes isomer-dependent oxidative stress and elevated C-reactive protein: a potential link to fatty acid-induced insulin resistance. *Circulation* 106 (15): 1925–1929.

Riserus U, Vessby B, Arner P, Zethelius B. 2004. Supplementation with trans-10, cis-12-conjugated linoleic acid induces hyperproinsulinaemia in obese men: close association with impaired insulin sensitivity. *Diabetologia* 47 (6): 1016–1019.

Saker ML, Jungblut AD, Neilan BA, Rawn DF, Vasconcelos VM. 2005. Detection of microcystin synthetase genes in health food supplements containing the freshwater cyanobacterium Aphanizomenon flos-aquae. *Toxicon* 46 (5): 555–562.

Sanchez W, Maple JT, Burgart LJ, Kamath PS. 2006. Severe hepatotoxicity associated with use of a dietary supplement containing usnic acid. *Mayo Clin Proc* 81 (4): 541–544.

Saper RB, Eisenberg DM, Phillips RS. 2004. Common dietary supplements for weight loss. *Am Fam Physician* 70 (9): 1731–1738.

Sewram V, De Stefani E, Brennan P, Boffetta P. 2003. Mate consumption and the risk of squamous cell esophageal cancer in Uruguay. *Cancer Epidemiol Biomarkers Prev* 12 (6): 508–513.

Shanmugasundaram ER, Gopinath KL, Radha Shanmugasundaram K, Rajendran VM. 1990. Possible regeneration of the islets of Langerhans in streptozotocin-diabetic rats given Gymnema sylvestre leaf extracts. *J Ethnopharmacol* 30 (3): 265–279.

Shigematsu N, Asano R, Shimosaka M, Okazaki M. 2001. Effect of administration with the extract of Gymnema sylvestre R. Br leaves on lipid metabolism in rats. *Biol Pharm Bull* 24 (6): 713–717.

Smedman A, Basu S, Jovinge S, Fredrikson GN, Vessby B. 2005. Conjugated linoleic acid increased C-reactive protein in human subjects. *Br J Nutr* 94 (5): 791–795.

Szapary PO, Wolfe ML, Bloedon LT, et al. 2003. Guggulipid for the treatment of hyper-cholesterolemia: a randomized controlled trial. *JAMA* 290 (6): 765–772.

Takekoshi H, Suzuki G, Chubachi H, Nakano M. 2005. Effect of Chlorella pyrenoidosa on fecal excretion and liver accumulation of polychlorinated dibenzo-p-dioxin in mice. *Chemosphere* 59 (2): 297–304.

Taylor JS, Williams SR, Rhys R, James P, Frenneaux MP. 2006. Conjugated linoleic acid impairs endothelial function. *Arterioscler Thromb Vasc Biol* 26 (2): 307–312.

Ulbricht C, Basch E, Szapary P, et al. 2005. Guggul for hyperlipidemia: a review by the Natural Standard Research Collaboration. *Complement Ther Med* 13 (4): 279–290.

Van Loon LJ, Van Rooijen JJ, Niesen B, et al. 2000. Effects of acute (-)-hydroxycitrate sup-plementation on substrate metabolism at rest and during exercise in humans. *Am J Clin Nutr* 72 (6): 1445–1450.

Villani RG, Gannon J, Self M, Rich PA. 2000. L-Carnitine supplementation combined with aerobic training does not promote weight loss in moderately obese women. *Int J Sport Nutr Exer Metab* 10 (2): 199–207.

Volpe SL, Huang HW, Larpadisorn K, Lesser II. 2001. Effect of chromium supplemen-tation and exercise on body composition, resting metabolic rate and selected biochem-ical parameters in moderately obese women following an exercise program. *J Am Coll Nutr* 20 (4): 293–306.

Index

beans, 82
  black-eyed pea stew, 201–202
  jicama sticks with roasted red
    pepper-white bean dip,
    219–220
  and pumpkin soup with chicken,
    black, 196–197
  as source of soluble fiber, 65
  vegetarian chili, 206
beef
  grass-fed, 54
  tenderloin salad, grilled, 207
  tenderloin scalloppini, 213
Beef Tenderloin Scalloppini, 213
beets, 49, 50
  recipes using, 209–210
Berry Smoothie, 195
beta-carotene, 50, 83
beta-glucuronidase, 67
betaine, 49
bile, 17, 60
  formation of gallstones from, 19
  importance of, 18
  release of, 73
  thickening of, 19, 72
binge eating disorder, 160
bingeing, 22
bioflavonoids, 50
bisphenol-A, 29, 34
bitter melon, 175
bitter orange, 177–178
Black Bean and Pumpkin Soup with
    Chicken, 196–197
black beans, 196–197, 201–202
Black-Eyed Pea Stew, 201–202
black tea, 98
  main difference between green tea
    and, 99
blood sugar
  balance, released toxins disrupting,
    34
  determining impact on, with glycemic
    index, 79
  fluctuations, 162
  increase of, 89
  lowering, 153
  maintaining stable, 64
  regulation of, 16–17
  rush, 21
  stabilizing, 83

blueberries, 49
  blueberry flax cereal, 195
  blueberry granola crisp, 224–225
Blueberry Flax Cereal, 195
Blueberry Granola Crisp, 224–225
blue-green algae, 184
body mass index (BMI), 35
  calculator, 35
Boston fern, 166
bottled water, 70
bottom-feeders, 58. *See also* fish;
    seafood
breakfast recipes, 189–196
breathing techniques, 160–161
Broccolini, 214
broccoli sprouts, 47
brown rice, 81, 83
  with kale, 206
Brown Rice with Kale, 206
Brussels Sprouts Soup, 199
buckwheat, 81

cadmium, 30
caffeine
  addiction, 98
  content in coffee, 102
  cutting back on, 97–98
  in green tea, 98
  in guarana, 178
caffeoylquinic acids, 65
cancer, 63
  -fighting compounds, 62
  prevention, 47, 53, 99, 183
  reducing risk of, 48, 154
Candied Sweet Potato, 192–193
caprylic acid, 181–182
Caralluma fimbriata, 176
carbohydrates, 65, 78
  continuous eating/bingeing on, 22
  conversion of excess, 17
  eating right, 78
  "good" and "bad," 78–80
  metabolism of, 17
  refined, processed, 162
cardamom, 58
carnitine, 53–54
Carob Mac Nut Drops, 223
carob powder, 65–66
carotenoids, 50
  fruits and vegetables containing, 51

7/11   ⑩   6/11
10/14 — ⑮   7/14
9/15
1/17   ⑰   5/16